TOP TEN BEST-EVER HEALTHY

WEIGHT-LOSS TIPS

ELLE ERIKSSON, RHN

iUniverse LLC
Bloomington

TOP TEN BEST-EVER HEALTHY WEIGHT-LOSS TIPS

iUniverse books may be ordered through booksellers or by contacting:

iUniverse LLC
1663 Liberty Drive
Bloomington, IN 47403
www.iuniverse.com
1-800-Authors (1-800-288-4677)

ISBN: 978-1-4917-1778-3 (sc)
ISBN: 978-1-4917-1779-0 (hc)
ISBN: 978-1-4917-1780-6 (e)

Library of Congress Control Number: 2013923529

Printed in the United States of America.

iUniverse rev. date: 05/19/2014

CONTENTS

ACKNOWLEDGMENTS

Thanks to my teenagers, Hannah and Josef, for not minding (seemingly) as I took some time to work on this project while you quite happily did your own thing. Thanks to Mom for supporting me in any way you could. I am pleased to finally present you with this finished product. (It may be small but it didn't happen overnight.) Thank you, Lisa Mabee. By helping me a great deal with the editing of the other nutrition/meal-planning cookbook (due at a later date), you've also helped me find my way with this one. Gratitude to all family and friends who were willing to cheer me on, lend your ears, offer valuable feedback, and patiently put up with me while I shifted some of my focus in order to see this little book to completion. I think you know who you are.

Thanks to my expert editor/advisor, Julia O'Loughlin. You were a godsend, *really*. You were able to wear a whole variety of hats as needed; a few more than you were expecting when you signed on. To Judy Koren, heartfelt thanks for being the voice of reason and rescuing me from that place of "not knowing when it's finished" and for final editing—like the experienced pro that you are.

My sincere appreciation goes to all who have led the way—the trailblazers: health-care professionals, researchers, scientists, nutritionists, environmentalists, writers, and other concerned citizens who have actively cared and continue to care so deeply about preserving and protecting human health, our food quality and supply, the welfare of animals, the environment, and our planet Earth.

A portion of the proceeds from this book will be donated to children's breakfast and lunch meal programs in local schools or areas where there is a need. The intention is to ensure that all children begin their day with delicious, nutritious, whole-food meals. The hope is that by giving children real food, and the nutrients that come with it, they will also receive comfort, growth, hope, and the ability to learn more efficiently. They will have a better chance of maintaining a healthy weight while taking the knowledge of nutrition and real food with them for life.

INTRODUCTION

My Story

My high-school and weight-gain years are long behind me, and I now have teenagers of my own, but I can easily recall what it felt like to gain teenage weight and how I did not care for it, not at all! It was quickly obvious to me that the trips to the donut shop with friends during school lunch breaks weren't working out too well for my formerly slender waistline. I clearly wasn't the only one unable to enjoy this deep-fried ring of sweet dough without the consequences of increased size and weight, but it seemed to me that I was the only one in my circle who was determined that this new, undesirable state of affairs was not to last. I was going to get back to and hold on to my slimmer side. It really mattered to me. Just wanting my pants to fit the same comfortable way they previously had seemed a good enough reason to begin with. The solution seemed simple, really. If poor food choices had gotten me into this mess, then avoiding them was going to get me out of it. There wasn't going to be "more of me to love" anytime soon! So I had to get smart fast, which was going to be easy, or so I thought.

I had been raised eating mostly food that was cultivated on our own land or at least homemade. We had a myriad of fruit and nut trees, berry bushes, a large vegetable garden, and lots of chickens. In the early years, we even had a dairy cow and a few goats that supplied us with milk from which we made cheese, butter, and ice cream. We never had access to the bags of Oreos, Fudgee-Os, and potato chips that the neighbors had in their cupboards and enjoyed at will. I mustered up a big ol' dose of willpower and got down to work. I set out to trade in the donuts, chips, and chocolate bars for more nutritious choices until I reached my initial goal of losing twelve or so pounds. Extreme for a teenager, yes, but that was my plan, and it worked!

In addition to eating better, I also discovered the weight-loss wonders of ten-speed cycling. My bike transported me, more and more often, from where I lived on the outskirts of town to see my friends in the city. Each ride meant a minimum of ten miles round-trip and quickly became a social and weight-loss winning combination.

As time went by, continuing to put smart eating into practice became less than straightforward. I yo-yoed with back-and-forth weight loss and weight gain while trying to figure out a sustainable, healthy way of eating. I also became aware that as soon as I could no longer eat just anything I wanted—without weight gain—I desired even more of it than I had before. Where did moderation go? Out the window, that's where! The emotional eating, the boredom eating, and the "it just tastes so darn good" eating continued despite my best efforts. I developed a long-term, on-again/off-again, unhealthy, dependent relationship with chocolate that would eventually need to be abandoned. I instinctively knew that the right path to take was the one leading me "back to the garden," even though following that path would be easier if all those tasty hindrances weren't there to block my steps. Luckily I also enjoyed healthy eating and conscientiously ventured further away from the sweets and eating swings. As a consequence, the mood swings, the energy swings, and the burden of extra weight that accompanied my poor eating habits and food choices subsided. I was well on my way toward a real-food diet and improved overall well-being. By the time I was ready to start my own family, I had established a nourishing whole-foods way of eating and had achieved a steady, healthy weight.

Knowing what I know now, I am actually grateful for my teenage weight gain because it motivated me to make healthier diet choices. I learned at an early age how integral a healthy diet is to general health and well-being and have continued to reap the benefits during my adult years. Many of my friends and peers are learning these lessons only now. Eventually poor diet choices will catch up with us all, regardless of how well our metabolism may have worked in our youth or early adulthood. And of course, in the end, healthy eating is not just about weight loss. It's really about benefiting from the multitude of other life-giving and disease-preventing bonuses that naturally stem from healthily pursuing your own ideal weight.

Having learned the fundamental importance and effectiveness of eating whole foods and engaging in physical activity, I have sought to spread my knowledge and help others struggling to attain their ideal body weight. Following my teen years, I took both fitness and fitness instructor courses, eventually studying nutrition and becoming a nutritional consultant and a cooking instructor. My personal journey and professional experiences have taught me which weight-loss techniques work and which don't. This book contains the ten strategies for weight loss that I have found to be most effective.

I'm not here to say that it's all about being slim, as we're fortunately now more able to accept and appreciate all body types and shapes. Instead, it is truly about finding a healthy weight, one that feels right underneath your layer of skin. The preindulgence weight, if you will: that place where you end and before the donuts start. This will naturally look different and be different on the scale for each individual.

Quite frankly, there is no quick fix. But there is a sustainable and successful fix involving a healthy whole-foods diet and an active lifestyle. Real food plus activity! It doesn't get much simpler than that.

A Note to the Reader

It is my hope that these top ten best-ever healthy weight-loss tips will serve as easy and sensible pointers as you travel along the path leading to the *you* you've been looking for.

The tips do not appear in any particular order of importance. Some discuss *what* to eat, while others discuss *how* to eat so as to improve important functions like blood-sugar balance and digestion. Obviously, what you choose to put into your shopping cart, order at restaurants, and ultimately put into your mouth is of the utmost importance to weight loss and good health. That being said, food choice is only part of the big weight-loss picture.

My suggestion is that you read through the book, assess which tips would be easiest or most realistic for *you* to follow, and then commit to only a few of them at one time. Keep in mind that, because we are all unique, something that seems to work well for one person may affect another person differently. For example, I was recently speaking with a woman who told me that, for her, cutting back on fats and oils was clearly the trick that directly and quickly impacted her weight. At the same time, a friend of hers found that reducing carbohydrates was undoubtedly her best ticket to dropping the unwanted baggage. Therefore, this book does not support any particular fad diet or all-or-nothing way of eating. The majority of diet books out there claim to be "the solution," offering one-size-fits-all weight loss for everyone while ignoring proven and effective strategies. From what I've seen, there is no *one* diet that is right for everyone's body. While a vegan diet may be best for one person, another person may decide that eating less grain and more meat is effective. People have a variety of personal preferences, convictions, and beliefs, as well as ethical, religious, geographical, and health-related reasons that determine the food choices they make. This book offers a more general approach to weight loss, with tips aimed at providing optimal results to anyone and everyone.

Immediately following the tips, you will find a 21-day journal designed to offer motivation and encouragement, as well as a place to plan, track, and record your progress.

Tip #1

KEEP YOUR FOOD COMBINATIONS SIMPLE

Take the load off a burdened digestive tract and refresh this dutiful servant with a diet that is simplified and purified. Weight loss is one of the many gifts of improved digestion.

The practice of creating simple food combinations not only improves digestion but also boosts energy and promotes weight loss. With this practice, meals are streamlined by separating food groups, primarily proteins from carbohydrates, because these groups digest at different speeds and utilize different digestive secretions. These differences can lead to competing processes within the digestive tract and may result in inefficiency and fatigue. Have you ever felt tired after a meat-and-potatoes meal? This digestive competition may be the reason. With a dinner meal that would normally consist of chicken, rice, and vegetables, try eating just the chicken (protein) and vegetables, designating the rice/grain (carbohydrate) for breakfast or lunch. Reduced busyness for the digestive tract equals more pep in your step.

When weight loss and improved digestion are achieved, you can return to a more complex meal, although it never hurts to add in a digestive enzyme supplement or a green salad with a meat-and-potatoes meal. But some people find that continuing to separate proteins and carbs at dinnertime not only helps their digestion but also prevents after-dinner low energy and helps them achieve a better night's sleep.

A few food-combining constants:

- Proteins and starches—carbohydrate-rich foods, including grains, breads, pastas, potatoes, and squash—are always consumed separately.
  Note: Vegetables and grains are both carbohydrates. However, unlike grains, vegetables do not convert to sugar (potatoes and other sweet and starchy veggies being the exception) and are therefore deemed neutral and may be eaten with anything, anywhere, and anytime.

- Fruit, drinks, or desserts should not be consumed with or after meals.

Why, you ask? Fruit naturally moves through your digestive tract very quickly, imparting its cleansing power, its energy, and its load of nutrients and fiber. But it requires a cleared pathway—an empty stomach—in order to accomplish this efficiently. Fruit consumed after a meal simply sits around on top of the meal in your stomach. Here it begins to spoil. This spoilage causes gas and bloating and interferes with the proper digestion of the rest of your meal. This is especially true for sizable meals that are high in protein, which takes longer to digest. Additionally, if you happen to have an overpopulation of bad or unhealthy bacteria in your digestive tract (a common problem), you'll be making their day, because they thrive (grow in numbers, by the billions) in this type of environment. For your digestive health, your general health, and your weight control, eating fruit after meals is a big no-no all around.

For these same reasons, fruit juice and any sugary drinks are also big troublemakers when included with meals. Additionally, liquids in general, including water, will dilute the potent digestive juices that are so necessary for the digestive tract to do its "breaking-it-all-down" work. The digestive process will be hindered. A sip or two of room-temperature or warm water is okay. Cold drinks, however, can halt the release of stomach acid (hydrochloric acid, or HCl), stopping digestion in its tracks. Then the subsequent chain of digestive events may also be interrupted. Drink most of your liquids between meals and limit your ingestion of liquids within half an hour of a meal.

Desserts are troublesome for the obvious reasons but are particularly perilous when eaten after a meal. Like fruit, they disrupt the digestive process of the meal you've just eaten, as the sugars begin mixing in, causing spoilage, putrefaction, and the release of toxins. To make matters worse, unless you have particularly healthy and robust digestion, the meal probably won't be moving along anytime soon. More time to rot. In such a case, you may find that the whole mess sets up camp, staying well into the night, wreaking havoc, and resulting in no sleep for you. Then you're left with the inevitable hangover—brain fog and lethargy in the morning. Next comes the convenience eating, and then come the sugar and coffee cravings. Oh, what a vicious cycle it is!

> *Can it be any mistake that STRESSED is*
> *DESSERTS spelled backward?—Unknown*

Although there are more food-combining rules, I've covered the ones that are most common and, in my view, most helpful for weight loss. Food combining is a relatively new technique designed for today's digestive systems as they face new challenges. Back in the day, people ate real food—nature-made, not tampered with, free from artificial and chemical additives, etc.—in sensible quantities. Unfortunately, this is too often not the case for many people today. Before the age of prescription and over-the-counter medications—both of which can also affect your digestive and intestinal condition and environment—most people likely had strong, healthy digestive systems better suited to handling more complex food combinations. This doesn't imply that everyone now has compromised digestion. Your body will usually let you know, in one way or another, if that's what you have. Your body is also capable of telling you whether you're either eating the wrong combinations of food or just simply eating the wrong food. Gas, bloating, chronic stomachaches, and feeling tired and heavy after a meal are just a few of the signs your body may use to inform you about its digestive challenges.

Despite this condition being relatively underdiagnosed, a reported one-quarter of US adults experience dyspepsia, a.k.a. indigestion.[1] Unfortunately, the hundreds of drugstore and natural products on the market aimed at bringing relief to symptoms of indigestion do nothing to address the root cause of the problem, so the relief is only temporary. This tip can help those who struggle with weight and/or digestive issues to attack the root of their problem. By not covering up the symptoms, they can address the true cause and achieve a long-term solution. (Tip #3 and Tip #5 also apply here.)

If you're not ready for food combining, at least keep your meals simple to improve their digestibility. Such a meal could include one protein, one carbohydrate, and some vegetables—for example, fish, rice, broccoli, and a green salad.

True Story

Robert, in his mid-forties, was advised by his doctor to lose fifteen to twenty pounds for the sake of his health. The plan was to keep him off the road that leads to high blood pressure, diabetes, and heart troubles. He loved food, had little self-control, and was developing a protruding belly. By practicing simple food-combining techniques and cutting out any unhealthy, high-calorie snacking, he dropped the weight in just six weeks. His pants fit him better and the storm in his stomach calmed down. He had more energy to draw on and was generally a happier and healthier guy.

Tip #2

BALANCE YOUR BLOOD SUGAR—LIMIT REFINED GRAINS, SUGARS, AND TRIPLE THREATS

Get ready, this is a biggie! Let's start with grains.

Opting for whole grains in place of refined grains is vital to making your weight-loss goals a reality. When grain (e.g., wheat) is refined (e.g., white flour), it is substantially stripped of nutrients like vitamins, minerals, fiber, and oil. Typically, commercial cookies, muffins, donuts, cakes, crackers, white breads, buns, and bagels are not only high in unhealthy fat and refined sugar but also contain mostly white flour. A triple threat!

All grains (carbohydrates) eventually break down into sugar. This may sound bad and cause you to wonder why anyone would eat grain, whole or refined, at all. The truth is, contrary to popular belief, sugar is not the devil. Sugar is actually fuel. Just as a car requires gas to operate, you require sugar. But before you go out and eat a chocolate donut for fuel, there's a bit more to the sugar story that you need to hear.

There are good and bad sugars. The good ones give you energy, whereas the bad ones deplete you of energy. The difference between good and bad sources of sugar lies almost entirely in how quickly they are absorbed into the bloodstream. Refined grain, existing in the most basic or simple form a carbohydrate can take, converts to sugar almost immediately in the body. With no digestive breakdown required, sugar is dumped into your bloodstream all at once. The result is high blood sugar, a.k.a. a blood-sugar spike.

5

Although the immediate results may be pleasurable, the inevitable blood-sugar drop that follows is not pleasurable in the least. Symptoms include fatigue, low mood, irritability, anxiety, sugar cravings, and coffee cravings, just to name a few. Sound familiar? And if that's not enough scary symptom news, here's the weight-gain clincher. People who regularly consume refined grain (unless they're *very* active and/or burn off energy at a high metabolic rate) consume more energy than their bodies can utilize. Simply put, unused energy is stored as fat.

Whole grains, in contrast, contain vitamins and fiber (in the outer layer) and oils (in the germ) and exist in a complex structure. Whole grains, therefore, take longer to break down and digest. As a result, they release their energy gradually, in sensible doses, keeping it and you going longer. With the slower release, the body has a better chance of using the energy up, not storing it as fat, and remains satisfied longer. With refined-grain consumption, you soon find yourself requiring another dose of quick energy (sugar) after the crash. This is where cravings and reaching for the sweet, refined, and convenient snack or treat (chocolate bar, donut, scone, cake, etc.) enter the picture. And so the cycle continues.

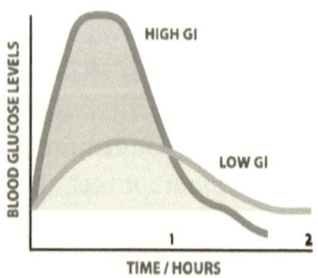

As the above graph shows, the higher blood sugar spikes, the lower it will inevitably plummet. To compensate for a spike in blood sugar, the body produces excess insulin that, after a short time, causes low blood sugar. Then the associated symptoms kick in, including more sugar cravings. If we heed those cravings, we send blood sugar back up. Then comes the inevitable plummet, hence the common roller-coaster effect of energy highs and lows that many of us experience on a daily basis.

True Story

Linda, a middle-aged friend who had been on the heavier side most of her adult life, with a few new pounds joining the journey each year, visited her doctor recently. The diagnosis was high blood pressure. She was also informed that she was obese and needed to lose twenty pounds. Her doctor advised her to eat whole grains, nothing white and refined in her diet. She already knew this to be a wise idea, but she really loved white bread and pasta. Although she wasn't pleased with the additional pounds over the years, she had previously said that she was simply bigger boned and was taking after her mother, accepting her weight as genetically determined. That was until the visit to the doctor. Thanks to the high-blood-pressure scare, Linda dived right into the new way of eating, and the pounds started falling off. "There is no turning back," she said. "I've never felt so good." She has actually also come to love the whole grains and has subsequently begun disappearing on us. I tell her, "Linda, we're losing you. You're missing part of your arms, but it suits you, you look great."

> *How can a nation be great if its bread tastes like Kleenex?*—*Julia Child*

Now let's take a closer look at how the body achieves blood-sugar balance. As you eat, your pancreas is constantly releasing insulin. This is the hormone responsible for regulating the amount of sugar in your blood. When your cells require more energy, insulin helps sugar (energy) to enter your cells.

If this doesn't happen, you die. When you too regularly intake more energy than your body can use, you enter into a state of perpetual high blood sugar. In time, the insulin receptors in your cells become tired of this constant battle and cease proper functioning. As a result, the body's ability to regulate blood-sugar levels can become less efficient. This condition is called insulin resistance and is the start of metabolic syndrome (previously known as syndrome x), the precursor to type 2 diabetes.

There is much more that your body must do to bring about the proper balance of glucose in your blood, but in a few words, when things get this far out of hand and you regularly have too much insulin (a fat-storing hormone) in your bloodstream, you begin to gain weight, especially in the midsection. What's more, it is believed that increased body fat makes it harder for the body to use insulin in the correct way. It's fair to say that when you reach this place, health and circulatory trouble (e.g., heart disease and hypertension) and other diseases like diabetes can be waiting right around the corner.

When it comes to grains, opt for brown rice, spelt, barley, millet, quinoa, oats, buckwheat, kamut, amaranth, and whole wheat. Choose manufactured and baked products that list 100 percent whole grain and are low in sweeteners and bad fats. You can also eat fresh fruit for a nutritious, fibrous energy source.

If, however, after taking up this whole-grain regimen you find weight loss unsuccessful (assuming you're not scarfing down ice cream and chips), you could try eliminating grain altogether for a few weeks, just to see what happens. Some nutritional pundits believe that for some people, any grain can be responsible for weight gain or difficulties with weight loss. For some, eliminating all grain may be worth a try, especially at dinnertime. Your diet will then consist of a good range of proteins—legumes, nuts and seeds, and lean animal products—plus fruits and vegetables. Another option is to first try substituting some of the other available grains for those you are currently eating. Remember that diversity is important and that each person is digestively unique. Everyone needs to figure out what works best for his or her own body.

Note: In the absence of carbohydrates, the body will convert protein (or fat) into energy. While this may sound good, it doesn't mean you should regularly depend on protein for energy. Here's why. The body's first priority is drawing energy from food. Low-carb/high-protein diets force the body to use a different method of transforming protein into available energy. Carried out long-term, this method is not recommended because it can create its own set of health problems.[2] In the case of extreme food restriction, the body will go so far as to convert muscle into energy for survival, a.k.a. wasting away.

Carbohydrates are also vital when it comes to mood balance. A lot of people don't know that depression is one of the most common symptoms associated with strict avoidance of carbohydrates. For many, their appetite can increase when they become depressed or are dealing with lowered mood. All of a sudden, as is so often the case, a dieting strategy can send them right back into the emotional eating pattern that got them into this mess in the first place.

Okay, let's move on to the sweet stuff. You now know about the problems associated with eating refined grains, which don't even taste sweet, so you can imagine what the sweet-tasting stuff does to your weight and overall health! Chocolate bar manufacturers want you to believe that their products are the answer to all your energy needs. It's true that they would be an answer if you asked, "What kind of snack should I choose for increased weight, dysglycemia (high/low blood sugar), and insane cravings?" The same applies to other triple threats like refined bakery goods—danishes, cookies, muffins, donuts, cakes, etc.—and many breakfast cereals.

True Story

> James, a thirty-six-year-old graphic designer, would regularly pick up a breakfast muffin and coffee while heading off to work. Without fail his energy crashed at 11:00 a.m. on the dot. His wife finally pinned him down at home for a breakfast of oatmeal with nuts, raisins, and a little honey. James soon noticed that his morning energy level increased and sustained until one o'clock in the afternoon without the crash. He also had better bowel function and within a month had lost ten pounds!

As far as desserts are concerned, when you're trying to lose weight, it's a good idea to "just say no." Your body surely doesn't need those extra hits of sugars and poor-quality fats, which give desserts their high count of empty calories. These treats are simply not worth it. Guilt quickly creeps in, the temporary pleasure vanishes, and your weight-loss goal is pushed further away while you maintain the vicious and addictive cycle of eating sugar. The more you have, the more you want! When you reach your goal, you can have an occasional treat with impunity.

If you need something sweet to taste without adding more inches to your waist, have a piece of fresh fruit or enjoy a small bowl of berries, which give an added bonus of vitamins, antioxidants, and fiber. Or satisfy your sweet tooth with a *few* pieces of dried fruit, such as figs, apricots, prunes, apples, or raisins. They're plenty sweet and natural, plus they provide a good dose of fiber and minerals. When using sweeteners, whether in coffee, tea, or baking, choose from whole-foods varieties such as honey, pure maple syrup, brown rice syrup, molasses, date sugar, sucanat, green stevia, and/or xylitol. These unrefined sweet sources impart valuable nutrients, which help your body handle these sources more sensibly.

But again, if you're going to partake of the sweets, you've got to go lightly, out of concern for both your weight and your overall health.

If you do consume the occasional baked good, eat only a small portion from a manufacturer whose products are just lightly sweetened (from dates, honey, unrefined sugar, or the other above-mentioned varieties) and contain only small amounts of healthy fats and oils (butter or coconut oil). Baking your own is the best idea. Moderate servings of healthy baked goods as an occasional reward will satisfy your sweet needs and give you that pick-up without doing damage. Fresh or frozen homemade fruit smoothies and slushies are also a real treat. They're low-cal, delicious, and good for you.

Steer clear of high-fructose corn syrup (HFCS). This blacklisted but highly used (and highly processed) product derived from corn has recently been spotlighted as a big contributor to obesity. It is sweeter and cheaper than sugar, which accounts for its extensive use in processed and packaged foods. Recent research suggests that it may be responsible for causing a specific type of weight gain that can be very difficult to lose.[3] The body can't process HFCS in the same way it processes natural sweet sources, and therefore HFCS is quickly and easily stored as fat. Once stored, it is difficult to convert back for energy use. Yikes! Beware of this one. It's also called corn syrup or glucose/fructose syrup, and it may show up in pop, candies, sports or energy drinks, fruit beverages, chocolate bars, jam, cereal, granola bars, yogurt, and all sorts of other packaged foods. It can even sneak into products that claim they're made with real fruit. Read labels and keep this villain out of the shopping cart.

Note: Artificial chemical sweeteners are not the answer to healthy weight loss—hence the words "artificial" and "chemical." Common (yet largely unacknowledged) symptoms related to artificial-sweetener intake include headaches, insomnia, memory loss, mood changes, abdominal pain, fatigue, joint pain, and skin imbalances (hives, rashes, etc.).[4]

The road to success is dotted with many
tempting parking places.—Unknown

True Story

Carla, a forty-year-old mother of three, had been carrying twenty-five extra pounds of fat around with her since her early twenties. She was fairly sedentary on weekdays because she worked in an office and spent most of her time at a desk. She would often go to the gym after work but never managed to shed the extra pounds she longed to lose. When she finally addressed her diet, making nutritious choices and cutting out the baked goods (particularly cake), her weight dropped steadily until she reached her ideal size. She then decided to treat herself once a week, on Fridays, to whichever coffee shop piece of cake she desired, getting back to business Saturday to Thursday. She remains slim and trim and maintains a wide smile of satisfaction.

Note: I haven't reached my tip on fats yet, but because this tip is all about sugar I need to share this with you now. Don't be fooled by "fat-free" labeling! Such labeling might as well translate to "no fat/low fat = high sugar = weight gain." For instance, consuming a refined grain product such as white rice crackers or rice cakes, even those that are free of added fat and sugar, will still result in conversion to sugar and then storage as fat if you take in more of it than your body can use. You need some fat/oil with the grains to slow the release of sugar into the bloodstream (whole grain comes with the oil built in). And as you will soon learn, you need fats for plenty of other reasons. But you must make sure to use only the right fats and in only very moderate quantities.

I was definitely one of those people who fell for the fat-free cookies and chips that are loaded with sugar and calories.—Alison Sweeney

CHEW YOUR FOOD AND BOOST THE ENZYMES

One of the most overlooked factors when it comes to weight management is the functioning of the digestive system. The digestive system is responsible for making food (its nutrients) available and absorbable in the body. There are many obvious reasons why you need these nutrients, but here's another weight-loss-friendly reason: Nutrients leave your body more satisfied, lowering the potential for lingering cravings. Furthermore, if you eat something that doesn't get digested, it is either stored or it increases your body's level of toxicity as your digestive system attempts to digest it. This level then needs to be lowered. In addition to food combining (see Tip #1), two of the best ways to get your digestive system functioning better are to chew your food thoroughly and to increase your consumption of enzymes.

So chew, chew, chew your food! Saliva is stimulated by the chewing action and in turn produces the alkaline enzyme called amylase, the big kahuna for carbohydrate breakdown. With enough chewing, your carbs can be well on their way to being digested before they even reach your stomach. Proteins also become much easier to break down after a jolly good pulverizing from the teeth.

Some experts say to chew each mouthful thirty-five to fifty times (whatever the food), while others suggest even higher numbers (if you can believe it), although it makes sense that some foods simply require less chewing than others. The goal is to literally transform the food into mush. These chew counts may sound unreasonable to you, but after a little concerted effort you'll likely get the hang of it, and increased chewing should become more realistic. After you get into the habit of chewing adequately, underchewing will simply feel wrong. However, well-cooked foods (e.g., vegetarian soups and cooked oats) and softer foods (e.g., yogurt and bananas) obviously just need to be chewed less than foods like almonds or steak. But why not give it a try to see how many chews seem right for you? Every extra chew counts.

Not only is sufficient chewing good for basic digestion, but it is also considered to be one of the most vital elements in weight management. When you take the time to chew sufficiently, you can focus on appreciating both the flavor and the meal itself. When you take longer to eat because you are actually chewing, your brain will receive the message sooner (often before you've finished the meal) that your stomach is becoming satisfied. Inevitably, less food is consumed, and that uncomfortable, "I'm too full" feeling is prevented.

An added bonus of a good chewing practice is better absorption of the nutrients in your food. It is very difficult for the small intestine to absorb large molecules of nutrients from food that is not properly broken down in your upper digestive tract (mouth and stomach). When food isn't broken down well, because of either poor chewing or faulty digestion, the evidence may appear in the fibrous and sometimes recognizable food bits that show up at the other end of the line. Proper chewing will help all systems extract more nutritive value from food. Chew, and your system will not be overtaxed. Postmeal indigestion will be reduced, and you'll feel ever so much better. Now you finally know why your mother told you to "chew your food."

True Story

My friend Heidi imagined that chewing her food more would be too difficult for her to start doing after decades of habitual underchewing. But still, she wanted to experiment with increased chewing. She actually found that it was not only possible but surprisingly easier than she had expected. She prefers the way she now feels after meals and can attest to the benefits of thorough chewing: relief from overeating, bloating, and indigestion, together with increased energy.

My Story

Since I've gotten into the habit of mindfully chewing my food well, I can now do it without even thinking or trying. It's become automatic, like breathing. Apart from an uncle who appears to have also taken to serious chewing, I think I chew more than anyone else I know. I am always the last to finish meals at family dinners. After all this chewing, I feel perfectly satisfied and don't even desire any of the dessert that is always served afterward.

Now let's move on to enzymes. Enzymes, which speed up digestion and metabolism, are available in raw foods, unpasteurized fermented foods (such as sauerkraut), and sprouted beans, grains, nuts, and seeds. These amazing little molecules may be the missing link in most weight-loss plans. Break down the food, take and use its goodness, move it out, and the weight drops off! As we age, our body's ability to produce enzymes, digestive and otherwise, diminishes. Each day, it may be that you start out with sufficient digestive enzymes, only to produce less or use up most of the production by the time dinner (often everyone's biggest meal) rolls around.

Here are a few ways to add extra enzymes to your meals:

- A spoonful of raw sauerkraut (fermented shredded cabbage) is packed full of digestive enzymes and healthy probiotics to help speed up and move along your dinner. If you've eaten more than your stomach is comfortable with, (say, at a buffet), try that spoonful or two of sauerkraut and the heavy feeling or discomfort of indigestion should soon lift. Sauerkraut can also be helpful for gas and bloating. Buy refrigerated, unpasteurized sauerkraut from a natural-foods grocery store.

- Raw vegetables, green salads, and fruit also have enzymes—the more fresh, the more enzymes. After produce is picked, its enzyme content diminishes steadily. Fresh herbs, such as parsley, basil, and cilantro, are also enzyme rich, so sprinkle them regularly on meals.

- When beans, nuts, seeds, and grains are sprouted, they are loaded with enzymes, not only making them easy to digest but also assisting with the digestion of the rest of the meal. Sprouting food increases its bio-availability—exposing more of its nutrients for easy absorption—in addition to neutralizing any anti-nutrients.

- Digestive enzymes in supplement form can be purchased from your health-food grocery store. Ask for advice and buy quality; you usually get what you pay for.

To make your own enzyme-rich, fermented, and cultured foods (e.g., pickles, vegetables, sauerkraut, yogurt, and more) and sprouts, check out the links below offering easy-to-follow recipes.

Your body will thank you. After all, enzymes are considered to be the fountain of youth.

- www.nourishingdays.com
- www.nourishedkitchen.com
- www.sprouting.com

Let food be thy medicine and medicine be thy food.—*Hippocrates*

True Story

One of my clients, Lauren, knows how careful she has to be with her food choices and how poorly she feels after most restaurant meals, or even after being invited for dinner at a friend's house. Vacations are worse yet, as too many days in a row of eating out and consuming different foods not only cause her all sorts of intestinal discomfort but also return her home with extra unwanted baggage—on her hips! She is sensitive to anything refined, rich, oily, and cheesy, such as meaty-cheesy lasagna, and often suffers after consuming these types of foods. Her sleep suffers, too, as the meal feels like it's still sitting there in her stomach partway through the night. I recommended that she purchase some raw sauerkraut, explaining how the additional enzymes would help the meal break down and travel through her system more quickly, not bogging her down. She promptly went out and purchased the sauerkraut, keeping it at the front of the fridge where she would more easily remember to use it. She has since been reaping the benefits of digestive comfort, even after those times of venturing away from home.

Tip #4

EAT HEALTHY FATS AND OILS AND AVOID HAZARDOUS ONES

Sorry guys, this one is a bit lengthy—it's a fat topic.

Contrary to the array of information that considers fat the enemy in anyone's battle to lose weight, our bodies do require some fat for good health and a healthy weight. Fats in meals also keep our bodies satiated longer and help stabilize blood-sugar levels. This helps to prevent between-meal snacking. But—and it's a big fat but—the right fats, and just a moderate amount of them, are what's essential. It's true that fats are especially high in calories. If you're trying to lose weight, go lightly and make your choices count. But also be aware that the numeric value of calories is not the whole story. When you consume calories from good sources, the result is energy for your body and for your metabolic processes. This is where the saying "we need fat to burn fat" comes from. When you consume calories from bad sources, there is no conversion to energy, and the result is flab and fatigue. Simply put, 500 calories of almonds or avocados will impact your body more beneficially than 500 calories of cookies. Quality trumps quantity.[5]

One of the healthiest categories of fat is the essential fatty acid (EFA) family. These are also termed omega-3 and omega-6 fatty acids. Because the body can't manufacture these oils, it is necessary, hence "essential," to obtain them from food. These EFAs help stimulate metabolic functions and are therefore a vital component in the maintenance of a normal and healthy weight. That's great news, but it's only the beginning. EFAs also improve the quality of skin and hair, enhance brain function, elevate mood (therefore preventing the comfort eating that may come with low mood), help balance hormones, and increase cellular integrity. Additionally, they are one of the keys to vitamin and mineral absorption. An adequate level of EFAs is essential to the homeostasis of the entire body.[6]

Because it's easier to obtain the omega-6 than the omega-3 fatty acid, extra effort should be made to consume foods or oils with a higher amount or ratio of omega-3. Great sources include fresh seeds (e.g., flax, hemp, pumpkin, sunflower, and chia) and walnuts, or the oils of all of these.

Note: The seed and nut oils listed above are polyunsaturated and unstable, meaning they can't handle exposure to light, heat, or air without becoming damaged or oxidized—oxidized equals production of free radicals, which equals cell damage in our bodies. Use them only in salad dressings and smoothies or by the teaspoon as a supplement, not in cooking. Buy your seeds and nuts fresh and raw and keep them refrigerated. Find the fresh flax- and hemp-seed oils in the refrigerator section of your natural-food store (check the expiration date and ensure that oils have been cold pressed). Polyunsaturated oils should be contained only in dark bottles to prevent light damage. Purchase oils from quality producers, such as Flora, Omega Nutrition, Udo's Oil, and Barlean's Organic Oils. Keep these oils refrigerated. If you're looking for a healthy oil supplement, Green Pasture makes an excellent product.

Other important sources of omega-3 fatty acids are fish such as wild salmon, mackerel, sardines, and herring, or their oils. Dark leafy greens also contain small amounts of omega-3, so you need to eat volume.

I suggest a salad of leafy greens and other vegetables (bell peppers, tomatoes, avocados, radishes, green onions, parsley, or dill), your choice of fresh seeds or nuts, goat-milk feta cheese, and a dressing consisting of one of the above-mentioned seed or nut oils, or extra-virgin olive oil, with fresh-squeezed lemon or lime juice, one crushed garlic clove, and unrefined sea salt and pepper. Toss and enjoy alongside a serving of baked wild salmon, mix in a cup of cooked (cooled) beans, or just go simple and eat it all on its own.

True Story

Allison, a twenty-nine-year-old mother of a toddler, was still hanging on to some of her postpregnancy weight. She switched to healthier oils as part of her strategy to lose the weight in a healthy way. She purchased a bottle of wild salmon oil capsules from the nearest health-food store and began taking the daily recommended dose. She lost the weight because she also made other healthy dietary changes and increased her physical exercise. However, the most notable difference since starting the wild salmon oil was how much more even her menstrual cycle-related moods became. She had previously been known for being particularly "hormonal" at these times.

More on fats and oils: Extra-virgin olive oil and sesame, avocado, canola,* and almond oils are recommended monounsaturated oils. They can handle medium temperatures (some higher) without becoming damaged. It's best to do a little research as their individual tolerance to heat varies. Look for the words "cold pressed" or "expeller pressed" to ensure lower manufacturing temperatures. Store these oils in a cool, dark place. Hazelnuts, pecans, almonds, sesame seeds, and avocados contain monounsaturated oil and are good sources of essential fatty acids.

Recommended fats that are safe for higher-heat cooking and baking are coconut oil and butter.

Coconut oil gets a blue ribbon for its superb abilities: It can raise body temperature, which in turn increases calorie

---

* Unless certified organic, most canola oil is derived from genetically modified crops.

burning—a process known as thermogenesis—and also contains fewer calories than other fats. Some people express concern that coconut oil is in the family of saturated fats and therefore may contribute to heart disease and all the other conditions associated with a diet high in fatty foods. But, contrary to popular belief, not all saturated fats are the same. Coconut oil is a medium-chained saturate. This means that the liver can break it down and convert it into energy more easily than would be the case for a long-chained saturate. Being readily usable by the body means coconut oil doesn't get stored as fat unless it is consumed in large amounts. Moreover, being a saturate, it is stable and therefore able to avoid the air/light/temperature pitfalls of the above-mentioned, unstable polyunsaturated oils. It is natural, edible, antifungal, and antibacterial. This oil can be a skin-care product, too.[7] Too good to be true? Apparently not! It seems to be a miracle oil, functioning as a great weight-loss oil and a health food. Buy quality unrefined coconut oil at your natural-foods or health-food store.

Beware of the fats and oils, hidden or obvious, lurking in many canned, packaged, and baked products. Avoid products that contain hydrogenated or partially hydrogenated oil. Oils listed as vegetable oil, which is commonly used in prepared, packaged foods and baked goods and found in restaurants (or sitting in your kitchen cupboard), can include soybean, canola, cottonseed, sunflower seed, safflower, or corn (and others). Most of these oils are also polyunsaturated, and, unless otherwise specified or when certified organic, the majority are most often derived from genetically modified (GM) crops. (For more on GMOs, including a possible weight-gain connection, see page 99.) The problem is that, because these polyunsaturated vegetable oils are unstable, they become damaged (oxidized, rancid) when exposed to air, light, and heat in refineries. During the manufacturing process, chemical solvents are used to extract the oils. These oils are then deodorized and bleached to remove any undesirable odor, appearance, and taste. Also removed are most of their antioxidants and beneficial plant chemicals.[8] As a result, these unnatural oils are toxic and, of course, hazardous to your health. When tampered with in this way, these oils become virtually indigestible and thus unusable by the body. I'm guessing you're starting to see a common theme in these tips; when the body can't use something you've ingested, this material is stored, not eliminated. Where is the most common and safest place for your body to store the unusable? You guessed it—in fat cells!

And just think how much worse it can get in the case of deep-fried food, where the same oil has been heated and used over and over again.

Nonhydrogenated vegetable oils are fine in moderation, provided they conform to superior manufacturing standards (e.g., expeller or cold pressed and/or organic). A big problem, however, is that we tend to get too much of these oils, leading to the same storage process discussed above.

One of the most dangerous fats to consume, and one, I might add, that will not help you lose weight, is margarine. You might not expect a nutritionist to tell you to replace your margarine with butter, but that's what I'm going to do! Margarine is 100 percent chemically based and factory processed. There is nothing natural about it and, therefore, not much in it to provide any benefit to your body. The chemicals and unusable fats contained in margarine cause that same storage-related increase and expansion in fat cells. Also worrisome is that margarine (and the other toxic oils) tend to overburden your liver. Tip #5 concerns this vital organ.

True Story

A few years ago, I visited a string of impoverished little towns located somewhere near the middle of Mexico's Baja Peninsula. I was informed that the native Mexicans residing there were known to have a somewhat shortened life span. They rarely lived long enough to reach the senior years. Many of them were also significantly overweight despite being poor. I also heard that the main cause of early death in these towns was heart disease. An American woman, who ran a day care for the children of some of these Mexican parents (many of whom were migrant field workers), had some insight into the matter. She told me that the women commonly used huge amounts of cheap, refined oil when cooking meals, often consisting of beans and white rice. It made her wonder if there was some kind of oil-heart disease connection. I checked out the local supermarket, and, sure enough, large containers of inexpensive corn oil and other vegetable oil blends were a main sale feature. I had dinner at the home of one of the Mexican residents and witnessed firsthand the excessive use of oil in preparing the bean-and-rice dish. It seemed to me that the beans and rice were cooked using a high amount of corn oil where one would normally use water or broth. The sad fact of the matter is that the vegetable oils commonly used by these people are high in polyunsaturated fat which means they're unstable. As a result they can easily become damaged (rancid) during the refining processes used in their production. Therefore, these oils pose a significant threat to heart health and also contribute to other health risks. These same oils are in widespread use in the rest of North America, so this is not a geographically limited health concern.

DETOXIFY! TAKE GOOD CARE OF YOUR LIVER AND REMOVE YOUR TRASH

Meet your lovely liver—the busiest organ in the body! Your liver is responsible for more than five hundred different functions. Its role in detoxification and fat metabolism are only two of the many reasons for giving thanks to and taking care of this incredible organ.

In addition to everyday pollution and toxins, our livers are burdened by prescription and other drugs, stress, junk food, chemical food additives, preservatives, and pesticides, unhealthy fats and oils, tobacco, and alcohol. Show your liver some love by avoiding these whenever possible. Remember, caring for your liver can actually lead to meeting your weight-loss goal.

Here is some much-needed assistance for the overburdened liver:

- Each morning, fifteen to thirty minutes before having food, coffee, tea, etc., squeeze the juice from half a lemon into a cup of warm or hot water and drink. This action provides a gentle daily cleanse for your liver and a wake-up for your gallbladder,* and it begins some

---

* Your gallbladder contains and distributes bile that is first produced by the liver. This bile emulsifies fat, breaking it down in preparation for its work, as needed, in the remaining digestive processes (i.e., the transport of vitamins and minerals).

intestinal tidying, a.k.a. house cleaning. As a bonus, it helps get your digestive juices flowing. These are all part of the solution in your pursuit of weight loss—and great health.

• Squeezing a lemon or lime wedge over your meal will help break down its fat content, rescuing the liver from having to do some of the intensive labor required for fat metabolism. This breakdown happens when lemon or lime juice is freshly added into oil-rich items like guacamole and hummus, or squeezed over cooked fish. Apple-cider vinegar from your health-food grocer also works well in place of lemon.

• You can also take chlorophyll supplementation in liquid form obtained from your health-food or natural-food store. Chlorophyll is amazing! Studies have shown that chlorophyll assists the body in detoxification; it even tackles heavy metals like mercury and neutralizes free radicals. Chlorophyll is alkalizing, nutrient rich, and energy boosting. It also possesses antioxidant, anti-inflammatory, and wound-healing properties. Chlorophyll serves as an internal deodorizer for your body and your breath[9] while feeding the good bacteria in your large intestine. Follow instructions and drink as recommended. Green powdered-drink formulations, such as those produced by Amazing Grass and Barlean's, also contain plenty of chlorophyll among their nutrient-dense ingredients. But you can also get your chlorophyll the old-fashioned way—straight from green vegetables (it's responsible for making them green). How's that for yet another really good reason to increase intake of those veggies? You can even juice your veggies. If you have a juicer, try adding kale or spinach and a little parsley to carrot/celery/apple juice or add the leafy greens to your blender concoction or smoothie. Perhaps you could supplement with the liquid chlorophyll or powdered green drink on those low-veggie days or when you feel you could use some additional detoxification and an increase of nutrients and energy. Some people add a few drops of liquid chlorophyll to each glass or container of water for steady, low-dose detoxifying and alkalizing throughout the day.

- Milk thistle, dandelion and dandelion root, burdock, and green tea are natural herbal products that can help cleanse and protect the liver, thereby improving liver health and function. You can purchase them in tincture, tea, or capsule form from your health-food or natural-food store. Consider adding fresh dandelion leaves to your salad or blending some matcha powder (stone-ground Japanese green-tea leaves) into your smoothie. **Note:** Be aware that dandelion is a diuretic, so drinking additional water is advisable.

- Beets, artichokes, cabbage, broccoli (cruciferous vegetables), onion, garlic, ginger, spirulina, chia seeds, and seaweed are also high on the list of foods that are helpful for clearing out toxins.

Kick out the trash! Regular bowel movements are a major part of weight loss and good health. You want total bowel evacuation at least once a day. Nothing should be left clinging to the sides of your colon, building up, narrowing the exit route, and damaging the intestinal walls. When damage does occur, diverticulitis, polyps, and colon cancer can develop. High-fiber diets are of utmost importance. Vegetables, fruits, whole grains, legumes, nuts, and seeds (including ground flaxseeds) are all excellent sources of dietary fiber, helping carry out your bodily waste, including toxins, LDL cholesterol, and all sorts of other impurities. Even circulating fat and excessive hormones (e.g., estrogen) are eliminated.[10] Unless these substances and the range of other impurities in our waste make it out in a complete and timely manner, they tend to reabsorb back into the bloodstream via the intestinal walls. They then require more detoxification by the already busy liver. Jeepers! That's enough to make a person sick!

Water, and plenty of it, is another major player in the detoxification process. Water helps to stimulate peristalsis—the wavelike action of your intestines that pushes matter through and eventually out of the body—and aids the kidneys to effectively perform their specialized detoxification work.

An elderly man told me that drinking two cups of warm water first thing in the morning brought him the "success that satisfies" early in the day. Some people rely on the caffeine kick in coffee to guarantee a morning movement. They might want to try the warm water first. Regular sleep cycles are also an aid to regularity.

I'm not gaining weight, I'm retaining food.—Author Unknown

It's beneficial to consume additional healthy bacteria, called probiotics or "friendly flora," in food or supplement form in order to improve bowel elimination. If you ingest too much of the sugar and alcohol that feed bad bacteria, use antibiotics that kill off both good and bad bacteria, or even drink chlorinated water (also a killer of both kinds of bacteria), you can easily throw your intestinal bacteria out of balance. Prescription drugs (including birth-control pills), intoxicants, stress, and poor diet can also upset bacteria balance. Many health problems can develop when imbalance occurs. Having a larger population of healthy bacteria greatly assists with waste removal and aids weight loss, in addition to being essential for overall good health. To replenish the probiotics in your large intestine, eat the unpasteurized sauerkraut (packed with healthy bacteria) mentioned in Tip #3. Other fermented foods, such as kefir, kimchi, and homemade fermented vegetables (e.g., cucumbers [pickles], beets, beans, radishes, carrots, etc.), also contain lots of good bacteria. Homemade yogurt is well cultured, and it, too, contains a large population of good bacteria. See the recipes in Tip #3 if you want to produce your own fermented vegetables or yogurt. Getting your probiotics has never been easier. You can now drink your friendly flora by choosing from the range of bottled, deliciously flavored kombucha tea drinks. Find them conveniently sold refrigerated and ready to consume at your local natural-foods store. Or try a quick and easy, healthy-bacteria repopulating regimen, using Bio-K+—a yogurt-like product, providing an intensely concentrated dose of probiotics in small single-serving refrigerated containers. Probiotic capsules are available in the refrigerated supplement section of the natural-foods store. Ask for assistance and buy quality. Human-strain probiotics are the most effective, but they are not as easy to find.

Although we haven't yet arrived at my exercise-related tip, remember that bowel and liver health are promoted by increased exercise. The sweat you produce helps your body to eliminate toxins, and the effort usually results in decreased stress. The liver benefits when stress is decreased because too much stress can create a toxic and acidic state within your body. As well, lowered stress usually leads to lowered use of unhealthy coping mechanisms and addictive substances such as alcohol, drugs, sugar, and salty, high-fat snacks—all of which are very hard on the liver. Additionally, regular exercise keeps not only you but also your bowels moving regularly.

True Story

Krista, in her early thirties and a stay-at-home mother of two young children, began experiencing poor health and increased abdominal fat because of a poor diet. She was a comfort-food eater who preferred a diet composed primarily of white rice, fatty chicken, bakery goods, chocolate, and minimal fruits and vegetables. She developed asthma, high blood pressure, allergies, constipation, and elevated levels of LDL blood cholesterol, all within just a few short years. She sought my advice about her undesired weight gain but was not yet willing to make the changes needed to achieve a healthy diet and lifestyle.

As time went on, her health condition worsened. Eventually, it became necessary to schedule an appointment with a cardiologist. She told me that she'd only be getting a call back from her doctor's office if there was a concern. The frightening call came, and she chose not to reply. Instead, she immediately began to apply the advice she had been given. She started eating brown rice (instead of white), lean chicken (forgoing the skin), and generous servings of vegetables and fruit. She turned her back on the box of chocolates and also began drinking more water.

Within days, she felt more energetic, and her bowels began to move regularly again. Over the next few weeks, she began dropping weight, her cholesterol and blood-pressure levels improved, the allergies subsided, and she was able to cut back on her asthma medication. She began to entertain the idea of walking and eventually did return the phone call. She felt great relief knowing she was finally on her way down the path leading to good health and a healthy weight.

Never look back unless you're planning to go that way.—Henry David Thoreau

Tip #6

MIND THE CALORIES— DON'T JUST COUNT THEM

Of course weight loss depends on taking in fewer calories than you burn. You already knew this! As discussed previously, this isn't as simple as "calories in/calories out." The important focus when it comes to calories should be on whether they are "full" or "empty." Most sauces, dips, spreads, and almost anything cheesy are loaded with bad fats and oils and will send your empty caloric intake skyrocketing in just a few bites. When you're trying to lose weight, avoid eating creamy or cheesy sauces or dips. Don't consume store-bought salad dressing, potato salad, and/or sandwiches laden with mayonnaise (egg salad, tuna salad). No bagels with cream cheese and no spinach dip allowed. Absolutely nothing battered and deep-fried allowed—ever! Obviously, cheesecake, ice cream, and chocolate bars are also on the hit list.

When eating donuts—only eat the center part.—Larry Wentz

Now, this doesn't mean that you should be restricting your diet so much that you find yourself starving and constantly unsatisfied by your meal. This lack of satisfaction is precisely why low-calorie dieting fails nearly 100 percent of the time. Willpower and discipline can only carry you so far. When making your food choices, consider nutrient density first and foremost. A feeling of satisfaction after eating is really important, but your diet choices must be healthy ones.

If you find yourself with limited options, perhaps when facing the appetizer selections at a party or when ordering a starter at a restaurant, choose something the body can appreciate and put to good use. For example, stick with items made from natural ingredients, like hummus or other bean dips, guacamole, black bean and tomato salsa, tzatziki, tapenade, or antipasto. Have them with a modest serving of whole-grain/organic corn tortilla chips or other whole-grain crispbreads, crackers or pita bread/chips, or use them as a dip for vegetables. If you spot items like smoked-salmon canapés, tomato bruschetta, kale chips, grilled vegetables, fish tacos, or meat or vegetable skewers/brochettes, or if you notice a seafood or sushi platter, then go ahead and enjoy a few pieces. Have a slice or two of cheese, if necessary, but generally take it really easy with cheese trays and stay away from anything deep-fried, sweet, or starchy.

Keep the following in mind when preparing or ordering foods:

- Meat should be broiled, baked, or grilled—never fried. Remove all possible fat.

- Great meal options include fish with a side of vegetables, vegetable-lentil or vegetable-chicken soup, vegetarian and meat chili, brown-rice sushi, bean/meat and veggie wraps (whole grain or lettuce), frittatas, and chicken or cashew vegetable stir fry. If serving a dish with rice or noodles, choose brown rice or whole-grain pasta.

- Have pesto or tomato-based sauces, rather than creamy sauces, on whole-grain pasta, rather than white-flour pasta.

- Use only a light layer of butter or coconut-oil spread on whole-grain toast or sandwiches. Try a thin layer of almond butter or another nut or seed butter.

- Use yogurt in dips and in salad sandwiches (egg, tuna, salmon, chicken) that normally contain mayonnaise.

- Eat a leafy green salad for a meal more often. Load it with fresh veggies and top with shrimp, chicken, or garbanzo beans and fresh nuts or seeds.

- Throw out any commercially made salad dressings. Make your own instead.

- Cut down on cooking oil in stir fries and sautés by partially replacing it with chicken or vegetable broth.

- Skimp on sweets! Instead of a typical dessert, make a low-cal fresh or frozen fruit smoothie or slushie in a blender. Use a little yogurt or your choice of milk (almond, rice, etc.) and a drizzle of pure maple syrup with your favorite fruit combination. Trust me, after enjoying a glassful you will not feel deprived or have lingering cravings. And remember not to drink these treats right after meals! Add a small handful of ground nuts or seeds or a spoon of nut butter and your smoothie can become a light meal. If you'd like a warm treat in fall or winter, cook sliced apples or pears in a saucepan in the juice from half a fresh orange; add a dash of cinnamon, a few raisins and pecans, and a drizzle of maple syrup. This mix is also excellent on oatmeal for breakfast or served over plain yogurt. An apple or berry crisp, low in sweetener and butter, is perfectly healthy and delicious. And nothing is so very wrong with an occasional piece or two of 70 percent dark chocolate as a well-deserved reward or at times when the going gets tough.

- Instead of pop (diet and regular) or juice, try sparkling water with a squeeze of lemon or a splash of juice. You can also choose a tasty herbal tea, such as raspberry or peach. Make a large batch of it and keep it in the fridge to replace your store-bought, sugar-laden juice.

When you eat a nutrient-dense, whole-foods diet—such as in the suggestions above or from the sites below—and go heavy on the vegetables and extra easy on the added cheese, oils, and sauces, you'll have no trouble feeling satisfied with your meals. This is where home cooking—from scratch—is really important. If you're concerned about calories, you'll be surprised with how much more food you're able to consume just to get to your daily recommended caloric total. Eating this way could make calorie counting a thing of the past.

See the following websites and blogs for plenty of delicious, nutritious recipe options and more food for thought: www .edibleperspective.com, www.wholefoodcooking.blogspot.com, www.mynewroots.org, www.cookieandkate.com, and www .loveoffood.ca.

For those of you who find that you're occasionally short on food-preparation time, it's a wise idea to maintain a stock of the healthier packaged goods, precisely for those rushed, stressful, no-time-to-cook days. As well, most health-food and whole-food grocery stores provide nutritious take-out or eat-in entrée selections, often freshly made, hot or cold, omnivore or herbivore, salad or entrée. These can be convenient, healthy, and time-saving options. When you purchase premade or packaged foods, always read ingredients with an eye for the red-flag items. You'll find a list of recommended brands and red-flag ingredients at the end of the book.

The elevator to success is out of order. You'll have to use the stairs . . . one step at a time.—Joe Girard

True Story

Melissa, a college student with a part-time job at a coffee shop, enjoyed a baked pastry and specialty coffee during each shift. Within two months of starting the job, she put on ten pounds of unwanted weight. Determined to turn her unhealthy weight crisis around, Melissa soon backed off and resisted the temptation of the baked treat and the syrupy coffee drinks that had become, for her, chocolate bars in a cup. She replaced these with healthy snacks from home and an occasional Americano or, more commonly, stuck to green-tea blends or chai tea with a little honey. She was able to quite quickly return to her pre-coffee-shop weight.

The reality is that most of us have bodies that succumb to this kind of treating as a regular occurrence. After a little investigation, I found out that many coffee-shop muffins, cookies, scones, and cakes hold from 350 to 450 empty calories, and that yummy mochachinos and the like can count in at between 250 and 400 empty calories, depending on size, extra syrups, whipped cream, etc. For someone who is trying to lose weight (or at least not gain it), this coffee-shop indulgence can account for almost half the daily suggested caloric total, minus the nutrients. It's a lose-lose situation.

Try to be satisfied most often with a cup of tea, chosen from the wide range of delicious blends also offered by these shops, and add a little honey if necessary. This drink totals zero calories without the honey, and about twenty calories with it. Otherwise, if coffee is a must have, try a single shot Americano or Swiss Water decaf, a little milk, and raw sugar or honey, or take it black for a total of five to ten calories. Half decaf/half caf is another option to consider.

Tip #7

EXERCISE AND BUILD MUSCLE MASS

Physical activity is crucial for weight loss and weight management. Additionally, next to having a healthy diet, getting adequate exercise is the most important factor in the prevention of the range of illnesses and diseases prevailing in our society today. Sleep is right up there, too, but let's just consider it a given.

Let's get started on this vital topic with an activity that needs little introduction and comes complete with a long list of compelling reasons for engaging in it.

Walking is an excellent form of physical fitness, within the capability of almost anyone, anytime, anywhere. It's easy, natural, and possibly the most effective activity you can do. Its benefits include weight loss, bone strengthening, improved digestion, and increased circulation. The additional oxygen you'll get from fresh-air intake during your walk will relieve stress, improve mental health, enhance physical energy, and provide you with an overall positive feeling. Regular walking can decrease high blood pressure and high blood cholesterol, improve cardiovascular health, deflect the onset of type 2 diabetes, reduce the risk of breast cancer in women, and help relieve chronic fatigue and fibromyalgia symptoms.[11]

Note: Women who walk regularly after being diagnosed with breast cancer have a 45 percent greater chance of survival than those who are inactive, according to a study published in the *Journal of Clinical Oncology.*[12] The researchers heading up the study also found that those who exercised in the year before being diagnosed were 30 percent more likely to survive compared to women who didn't exercise during the time leading up to their diagnosis.

What's more, walking boosts your immune system! Walking regularly can lower your risk of arthritis, macular degeneration, and even cancer by an astonishing 50 percent compared with people who don't exercise.[13]

Last, but not least—it only takes thirty minutes of brisk walking to burn off 150 calories!

> *Walking is the best possible exercise. Habituate*
> *yourself to walk very far.—Thomas Jefferson*

True Story

Michelle, a thirty-five-year-old high-school teacher, started a new job within walking distance of her home. She began walking to and from work every day, about sixty minutes in total. Within several months she had lost the fifteen pounds that had plagued her for years.

Moving right along and picking up the pace—if you're hoping to have your extra weight drop off faster or you're having trouble with that last stubborn layer sitting around your hips or abdomen—you may need to increase the cardio in order to "make it happen." You might even want to get the hard work out of the way early in the day. In a TV interview, actor Anne Hathaway was asked how she got slimmer and fitter for her Catwoman role in *Batman: The Dark Knight Rises* and slimmer yet for her character in *Les Misérables*. She said she took the advice of fellow actor Hugh Jackman, who told her of his method for firming up and shedding a layer. He said he'd jump on the treadmill first thing in the morning before he ate anything. This way his body was able to burn off fat more efficiently by converting it into needed energy. If he'd eaten first, his body would have had to burn through the calories of the food before reaching any fat to be burned. That's good advice when we need to get serious. Just make sure to eat nutrient-dense food afterward. Your body will put this food to some very good use.

If you're not already accustomed to cardiovascular or aerobic exercise, work your way up the cardio-intensity ladder gradually. Start slowly or exercise at a lower intensity for a longer duration. Remember, set realistic goals for yourself and keep reminding yourself that any bit of physical activity is better than sitting on your butt!

One of the lesser-known benefits of exercise is improved awareness of your body and its needs. After engaging in intense cardio activity at the start of the day (or later), you will not only reap the benefits of a good mood or "natural high" thanks to those cardio-induced, feel-good endorphins that kick in, but you'll also naturally set yourself up to make smart food choices for your body. Just think, it's pretty uncommon to see someone leave their gym or finish a jog and head straight for a fast-food restaurant or devour a chocolate bar. That's right! Your body will automatically seek the real thing.

And on that note, here's a further benefit: Physical exercise plus good nutrition help keep your joints in good condition— something you'll appreciate if you plan to continue exercising or doing anything else that requires movement.

More exciting and motivating news: Your metabolic rate stays elevated for several hours after cardiovascular and aerobic exercise, causing you to burn more calories even at rest.

Whether you do your cardio first thing in the morning or later in the day, make sure you "just do it." Jogging, cycling, rowing, and swimming are on the long list of cardio activities that are open to you. Gyms also offer a variety of great fitness classes. They are a fun way to slim down, get toned, firm up, "sweat out your junk" (mental and physical), and achieve balance. Try the classes out and find one or two that feel right for you. At community centers you can sign up for team sports like soccer or volleyball, find a dance class, or meet a tennis instructor or even a partner. Choose your preferred methods of cardio, decide where to do them (outdoors or indoors at the gym), and just do them, regularly, three to five times a week.

If you already know what to do, have the discipline and the motivation, and simply don't care for going to the gym, you can do it all at home, the way I sometimes do. I actually like the gym, but during the fair-weather months or for the sake of time or convenience, I work out from home using a combination of indoor/outdoor fitness, often starting with floor exercises, light weight lifting, or low-impact aerobics. To make it nice and easy, or at least more enjoyable, I do it to my favorite TV show. Even if you just watch the news or the Discovery Channel, you have a chance to get down and give yourself twenty and get your routine started. My guilty pleasure—*The Ellen DeGeneres Show*. I hardly know I'm working out! All too soon, my favorite show and my workout are finished.

A good comedy also brings me many welcome, stress-reducing laughs, adding years to my life. It even wakes up my abs. Push-ups, sit-ups, other abdominal work, lunges, and Pilates can all happen in your living room if you've got the discipline. Get a few light weights for your shoulders, back, biceps, and triceps. If you know any low-impact aerobics, you can do them too or put on some great tunes and dance up a storm, a fun weight-loss storm. "Burn baby burn, disco inferno!" Aerobics and dancing work your whole body, even those places that are hard for a walk, run, or cycle to reach. Next I put on some favorite music, and outside I go for a thirty- to forty-minute bike ride, light jog, or brisk walk (sometimes a combination of these). I always stretch out afterward. You want flexibility and long, lean muscles. I try to keep up with exercising three to five times a week. I don't usually go through my entire routine all in one day, and I always leave a couple of days in between working out a muscle group (e.g., abs or triceps), as muscles require time for repair. Sometimes I switch it up—perhaps by starting with cardio—or add something new, and when time is tight I make workouts shorter or at least get in a thirty-minute walk.

Keep in mind that the more you enjoy an exercise program, the more likely it is that you will continue to do it. Reflect on any type of activity that (a) is enjoyable and (b) requires activity (e.g., dancing, walking your dog, gardening). Anything will do as long as it gets you moving. Then consider that activity from the point of view of increasing the physical exertion it requires. If you walk your dog, how about taking your dog for a run? If you feel like you don't have time for exercise, think about how you might be able to slip it into your busy schedule alongside something you already have to do. For example, park or get off the bus farther away from work, school, or the market, or if possible, walk or cycle all the way there. Take the stairs instead of the elevator. If you have a yard, turn your yard work into exercise. When I had a good-sized yard, I'd make mowing the lawn, raking leaves, or digging up some land for the vegetable garden all count as a workout. For that matter, housework (e.g., washing floors, walls, or windows) can also double as body shape-up work.

Those who think they have no time for bodily exercise will sooner or later have to find time for illness.—Edward Stanley

True Story

Jessica, a twenty-three-year-old nursing student, put on extra pounds quickly from all the months of sitting, whether in class or at home (reading, writing papers, and studying for exams). Soon all of her pants had become too tight, and she felt terribly uncomfortable. Her previously active lifestyle had been put on hold as she focused on schoolwork and ate more snack and convenience foods than usual. Rather than shopping for bigger pants, Jessica got right back into her workout routine. She made it to the gym or went out for a jog several times a week. She soon dropped a size and steadily slid down to her preferred weight, simultaneously feeling great (even victorious).

Also True

Andrew, a fifty-year-old accountant, was having trouble losing a decade's worth of extra stubborn weight. It was when he finally began riding his bicycle to and from work—forty minutes each way—that he rapidly shed the extra pounds. His mental health also improved considerably. Additional bonuses included free transportation, no parking fees, zero environmental impact, increased physical and mental energy, and an improved overall state of health.

Weight training is also very helpful for reducing body fat.[14] Why? Because muscle burns off fat! The more muscle, the more fat-burn-off potential. Building muscle, the body's recovery from doing so, and simply having muscle mass all consume additional energy and boost your metabolism. That's incredible! It means that if you possess an adequate amount of muscle, you're constantly burning off more energy than you would if that muscle weren't there. Ever heard of burning calories just by twiddling your thumbs? Well, it seems that, for the muscular, this too is possible.

A substantial amount of muscle is also beneficial for maintaining and supporting a healthy skeletal structure. As it is, you naturally lose muscle as you age, and because muscle loss precedes bone loss, it is important to build muscle around the bones and ensure you keep it there.[15] You should get started right away if you haven't done so already. It's easier to build muscle when you're relatively young and haven't yet hit those muscle-losing years. Luckily, muscle has memory, so even if you take a break from muscle building, when you start up again, your muscle will build back quickly. Don't wait too long, though; "use it or lose it" is no joke. And don't wait until you're too old and weak to lift anything heavier than a coffee cup—and your love handles have become as big as your saddle bags. It may seem like much too little almost too late. But the good news is that it's not! If you lose some weight, make smart food choices, and get moving, things can only get better.

Note: If you're new to weight training or muscle building, it's wise to seek instruction from a certified fitness trainer at your local gym, fitness studio, or health club.

Fitness: If it came in a bottle, everyone
would have a great body.—Cher

Tip #8

EAT LESS MEAT—MORE BEANS, PLEASE

Regular meat consumption is often linked to weight gain, whereas vegan (no animal products) diets are associated with a lower and healthier body weight.[16] I personally know only a few strict vegans, but I can tell you this: They're slim and they're looking pretty healthy. All over the TV, famous people are sharing their vegan stories, telling us that since going vegan, they have never felt better or had their weight drop faster. Everywhere we turn, we hear experts saying that we should all reduce our intake of meat and dairy and increase our consumption of plant-based protein sources such as legumes, nuts, and seeds, in addition to eating more vegetables and fruit.

One of the big bonuses of a plant-based diet is that it is a more alkaline-producing diet, while a meat- and animal-product-based diet is more acid producing. Many of us are now aware of the importance of a higher pH level (more alkaline than acid) in our body for disease prevention purposes, but higher alkaline levels are also crucial for weight loss. Because this is all happening at the cellular level, we need to be aware that the more acidic the cell, the more weight-gain potential it has.[17]

True Story

I was speaking to a fifty-five-year-old woman recently who revealed the secret to her weight-loss success. She had been trying different diets for years but never achieved the hoped-for results. It was her doctor who advised that she try switching to a diet higher in alkaline foods in order to help her lose some of her extra pounds. The weight loss came more easily and more quickly than she could have imagined. She lost seventeen quick pounds by cutting way back on meat and dairy, replacing them with plant-based protein foods, and significantly increasing her vegetable intake.

Meat also takes longer to digest than nonanimal protein sources. In some cases it moves along far too slowly, spoiling in your small intestine and causing damage to the colon. As you've already learned, regularity with total intestinal evacuation is one of the secrets of weight-loss success. Well-balanced vegan diets are associated with higher waste-removal ability and lower rates of heart disease, cancer, arthritis, diabetes, and a host of other ailments, including all the problems associated with chronic constipation.[18]

Let's take a closer look at the plant-based, animal-free protein options:

Nuts and seeds are a very nutritious protein source, but they need to be fresh or they become a health risk because of the rancidity of the oils. And remember, because nuts and seeds are high in oil, albeit healthy oil, you must consume them in moderation both for the sake of your weight and for the extra work for your liver (the organ in charge of fat metabolism). It's interesting to note that it is more difficult to binge or go nuts on healthy foods like almonds. Eat a whole bag of chips, sure, no problem! Eating a bag of almonds becomes a bit more difficult—unless these nuts are loaded with salt and drenched in extra oil or coated with chocolate—none of which is recommended. Because healthy foods, like nuts, are nutritionally balanced, they are very balancing to those who consume them. It is difficult to become addicted to them. We tend to become addicted to foods that are nutritionally void or unbalanced.

Legumes—which includes beans, lentils, peas, and others (but I'll mostly be calling them beans)—are the protein-rich, practically fat-free, nutritional powerhouses that most of us should be eating more often. Another benefit—they're cheap! Besides being very economical, they store well, don't require refrigeration (until cooked), and are not contaminated with *E. coli* or salmonella. Replacement of a meat-based diet regimen with a bean-based one has further ethical and practical implications. No living being (i.e., the meat source) needs to give up its life, and worries about listeria and mad-cow disease become things of the past. Beans are extraordinarily nutritious! They're packed full of vitamins, minerals, and disease-fighting phytochemicals, while being very high in fiber and low in carbs. There are many additional benefits—or shall I say "beanefits"—varying from bean to bean. Take the black bean, for example. It possesses properties known to be beneficial for blood, kidney, and reproductive health and can aid in the relief of lower-back and knee pain. Traditionally, the juice of the black bean is believed to help dissolve kidney stones, improve urinary difficulties, diminish hot flashes caused by menopause, and speed recovery from laryngitis.[19] Retain the bean cooking water and drink half a cup, half an hour before meals. And to think, all of this from just one bean.

Beans are beans and must not be confused with fake or mock meat products made primarily from isolated or concentrated soy protein. Some careless vegan diets rely on isolated soy protein to form the majority of protein intake. Soy protein is not a whole food, and from all that I have learned, it should be eaten only sparingly, if at all. The reality is, when you eat packaged or processed food, you're often ingesting a lot more processed soy than you realize.

Whole soybeans, edamame, and tofu are a better way to go if eating soy, although even these are best eaten only in moderation. Soy contains isoflavones, a form of phytoestrogen (a plantlike substance) that mimics estrogen in the body and can interfere with normal estrogen levels.[20] Soy is also high in phytates, also known as antinutrients, which block some mineral absorption.[21] In Asian countries where soy is famously eaten frequently and the rates of some cancers are reportedly low, the soy is still eaten only in small amounts and is usually in a fermented and more digestible form (tempeh, soy sauce, miso, fermented tofu, or sprouted soybeans). Some studies suggest that the low cancer rates (particularly for hormone-related cancers) may be more closely linked to the lack of dairy in most Asian diets rather than to regular soy intake.[22] Another important piece of information is that soy is the strongest of the goitrogenic foods, capable of producing a slowing-down effect on the thyroid gland.[23] The thyroid gland is responsible for producing hormones that regulate your body's metabolic rate.

The topic of soy is clearly controversial, and there is a lot of confusion about the potential health benefits and risks associated with soy. The truth is that soy itself is not necessarily the problem. The problems that have come to be associated with soy actually result from corporate food production or agribusiness (no surprise here). Industry has turned soy into a cheap commodity crop, which is most often processed, concentrated, and/or genetically modified.* Being cheap and plentiful, soy is used as a filler by the majority of companies producing processed and packaged goods. As a result, our population has become overexposed to this difficult-to-digest food. This overexposure has, in turn, contributed to an increase in allergies and sensitivities, not to mention the vast and varied symptoms (e.g., gas, bloating, diarrhea, and irritable bowel syndrome) related to digestive disorders.

---

* Unless certified organic or otherwise stated on the package, soybean and corn products most likely originate from genetically modified (GM) crops. Even products labeled organic are not guaranteed to be 100 percent GMO-free. Cross-contamination between crops is very common, and in many cases organic soybeans are found to be contaminated with GMO beans.[24] For more on GMOs see page 99.

The skinny, mighty, bountiful beans and other legumes I'm emphasizing here come in many varieties. These include black, navy, small white, lentils, mung, adzuki, cannellini, great northern, broad, pinto, lima, garbanzo (chickpeas), split peas, and black-eyed peas. There are so many ways to prepare all of these beans and enjoy the full range of styles and tastes. Thousands of simple and delicious recipes can be found on the web or in cookbooks. Put beans in chilis, quesadillas, wraps and rolls, dips, soups, and even brownies. You name it, beans are there for you. See the recipe websites mentioned in Tip #6 for some bean inspiration.

It is a well-known and widely experienced fact that beans can be gas producing, with many people finding them difficult to digest. Most of this difficulty can be remedied by following proper cooking methods. It is important to rinse and then soak dry beans overnight or for a day, in plenty (three to four times the volume) of water and a bit of apple-cider vinegar. After soaking, drain off the water and cook in fresh water. Bring to a boil, skimming off any foam that rises to the surface, lower the heat, cover and simmer until the beans are soft, then drain once cooked. Cooking time varies depending on the bean. This soaking/cooking method improves digestibility by removing the trisaccharides and phytic acid (the mineral-blocking compound contained in beans). Cooking beans with herbs and spices also helps to improve digestibility. Choose from anise, caraway, cardamom, cinnamon, coriander, dill, fennel, ginger, thyme, etc. Still, for the novice bean eater, the best policy is to ease your way into beans. Allow your body to get used to them slowly, as it will need time to gradually produce the breakdown enzymes that are required for good bean digestion.

Note: Other foods, like grains, nuts, and seeds, can also be soaked using the above method to remove the phytic acid or other antinutrients and increase the bio-availability of that particular food. However, only the grain would be cooked afterward, while the nuts or seeds would be eaten raw or oven-roasted at a very low temperature. Beans, grains, nuts, and seeds can also be sprouted to further increase the bioavailability of their nutrients and enzyme content. See Tip #3.

Although this tip has been mostly about including more beans and reducing the amount of meat in your diet, if you're not interested in becoming a vegan or can't imagine your life without meat, that's fine. No need to get extreme here. Try cutting your meat intake down to only one meat-containing meal per day or going meatless every second day. Or try being a weekday vegetarian and have meat, if you want it, on the weekends. For most people, these strategies would reduce meat intake by 50 to 70 percent.

> *You're thinking I'm one of those wise-ass vegetarians who is going to tell you that eating a few strips of bacon is bad for your health. I'm not. I say it's a free country and you should be able to kill yourself at any rate you choose, as long as your cold, dead body isn't blocking my driveway.—Scott Adams*

My Story

I am not a vegan but tend naturally to steer more in that direction. I'm not entirely convinced that we are all meant to follow that path, because people have eaten meat since practically forever. And some Arctic dwellers eat nothing but meat as a result of nothing else being available. Even some nonpolar people feel better when they do eat some animal protein. However, today's world presents us with other matters to consider. Much has changed in our "eating animals" world. There now exists a good (perhaps even an urgent) handful of reasons for reducing meat consumption. Aside from cutting back for health-related reasons, we may also choose to cut back for the sake of the environment. According to the Food and Agricultural Organization of the United Nations, more greenhouse gas results from the livestock industry (18 percent) than from all forms of transportation combined![25] An article in *The Guardian* (2012) based on a study published in *Environmental Research Letters* says, "Meat eaters in developed countries will have to eat a lot less meat, cutting consumption by 50 percent, to avoid the worst consequences of future climate change."[26] A related and compelling reason for reducing meat consumption is directly linked to concern for the welfare of the brutally treated animals raised on conventional livestock mega-farms. This combination of reasons has caused many a carnivore to consider where their meat comes from, to turn to sustainably raised animal products, and/or to reduce, or even cease, consumption.

Here are additional related reasons: The conventional livestock industry makes a huge contribution to polluted waterways, energy use, rainforest destruction, and land degradation; a tremendous amount of crops are grown specifically for animal feed; animals are drugged up, so the milk and meat are drugged up too (promoting antibiotic resistance, etc.); and inhumane conditions are imposed upon both animals and factory-farm workers. If you're a meat eater, think sustainable! Look for organic or free-range meats and dairy for a nonmedicated, more nutritious, earth-friendlier/animal-friendlier product. "Grass-fed" is another important term to look for because grass is the natural diet of grazing animals. Eating a natural diet improves the health of the animal and therefore improves the healthfulness of the meat or dairy you're eating. Grass-fed meat is much higher in omega-3 fatty acids as opposed to omega-6 fatty acids. The latter predominates in meat from animals fed corn or soy.

You are what you eat eats.—Michael Pollan, from
In Defense of Food: An Eater's Manifesto

When chickens get to live like chickens, they'll taste like chickens, too.—Michael Pollan, from The Omnivore's
Dilemma: A Natural History of Four Meals

Note: Organic and free-range products may be more expensive, but in light of all the above, I'd say they're worth it. And if you are willing to reduce use of animal products, substituting the more economical plant-based protein options, the cost should even out. Stock up your freezer when there's an organic meat sale, not only saving money and time but also reducing all those trips to the store. The price of animal products purchased directly from the local farms offering them can be significantly lower, and you can further reduce the price by buying in bulk.

Find more ethical and nutritious animal-based products at your local farmers' markets, natural-foods grocery store, or free-range farm (selling to the public). See the following website to find your nearest producer of grass-fed meats: eatwild.com /products/index.html. Read more on buying organic, fair trade, and local on page 97.

Fish is a great source of protein, but fish are also another matter of grave concern. As you may already know, several species of sea life are now extinct while many others are facing extinction because of destructive fishing practices and overexploitation. At the same time, oceans and lakes are becoming increasingly polluted. Still, if you choose to continue eating fish, I'd usually recommend wild as your best option, but first check the websites below and view their lists showing which fish are okay to enjoy and which to avoid. Also check which species of farmed fish and seafood are grown in a sustainable, responsible manner (i.e., in closed containment, with sustainable feed, and in proper locations), making them the better option over endangered or overfished wild fish/ seafood stocks. Be aware that some of the fish-farming industry (particularly salmon, using open-net pens) continues to be shown to have disastrously impacted not only specific ocean life but also whole ecosystems, including all kinds of bodies of water and the land animals and people relying on or eating from them. Additionally, the farmed fish's diet often includes animal by-products and GM corn and soy. At the time of writing this book, the GMO conglomerates are discussing and engineering a rapidly growing GM salmon. I don't know about you, but when I eat fish, I want to eat the real thing, not some genetically modified "frankenfish," nor a fish that was brought up in conditions mimicking the worst of the big factory-feeding operations, where huge numbers of cows, chickens, turkeys, and pigs live (and die) lives of suffering. For more information on the perils and impacts of open-net pen fish farming, I recommend the documentary *Salmon Confidential* (www .salmonconfidential.ca), where you will discover how our choices can help to either destroy or save an entire ecosystem.

Visit www.montereybayaquarium.org or www.oceanwise .ca to view the list of fish and other seafood that are "okay to eat" or are "not recommended." Also see www.greenpeace.org to discover how supermarkets are rated according to how they provide consumers with sustainable seafood.

As you can see, I have more than enough reasons for becoming vegan should I decide to go that route. In the meantime, while I journey the road of "eating less animals" and cook accordingly when feeding my kids (who still want some meat), I will continue to choose products that I know originate from animals raised with at least "farm to market" friendliness.

However your protein choice is directed—animal, vegan options, or a combination—consuming plenty of fresh vegetables and fruits, whole grains, and proteins from different sources maximizes the potential for your good health by making available a myriad of food nutrients. There is a direct tie here to weight management because a healthy body metabolizes nutrients most efficiently when presented with the whole spectrum of all the essential ingredients. Energy and efficiency up just naturally tends to lead to weight down.

Note: Vegans need to make an extra effort to consume both enough complete protein and enough foods containing sufficient levels of iron and vitamin B12. Some herbivores deem it necessary to become lacto-ovo vegetarians (include dairy and eggs) or even to include fish in their diet in order to combat iron and B12 deficiencies.

True Story

Kate and her husband, both working and raising their teenage girls, got busy and bogged down with various life necessities. Perhaps they even became a bit lazy. Food became fast, refined, meaty, and cheesy. Kate went from a size four to a size eight within two years. While on a cruise, she noticed that her companions had not let their bodies go the way she had. She asked me how she could reclaim the slim figure that once was hers. She was motivated and followed all my recommendations: Eat whole foods, exercise portion control, avoid extra nibbling, and reduce intake of meat and animal products. She also seized opportunities to get her body moving. She walked from A to B whenever possible and got busy in her small home gym a few times a week. Kate is now fit, firm, and fab after forty. The rest of her family also benefited from her careful shopping choices and more nutritious meals.

I'd never seen determination such as Kate had. It goes to show you that if you work at it hard enough, what can be yours will truly amaze you. What's required is commitment and effort. It's not always easy to get started, but after you stick with it awhile and begin to see those hoped-for results, it can get pretty exciting. Over time, everything connected with your diet and exercise program will become easier, and the results will accumulate.

When you get right down to the root of the meaning of the word succeed, you find that it simply means to follow through.—F. W. Nichols

Tip #9

CONSIDER CUTTING WHEAT AND/OR DAIRY

After meals, do you experience bloating, fatigue, and headaches? Have you gained weight for no apparent reason? The cause could be wheat and/or dairy.

Let's begin with wheat: Although many grains are commercially available, wheat is prized in food manufacturing and is used in about 95 percent of all store-bought baked goods, bread, pasta, etc. This is mainly because of its high gluten content, which makes it excellent for baking. You may have therefore unwittingly overeaten wheat (and gluten) and now experience symptoms like fatigue, bloating, and abdominal weight gain. Did you know that today's conventional wheat has been hybridized over and over so many times that it doesn't bear much resemblance to the original wheat kernels? The gluten content is said to be hundreds of times higher than that of precommercialized wheat.[27] This drastic alteration may explain a few things, one of which is the increased frequency of sensitivities and allergies to gluten.

Perhaps this news about wheat leaves you wondering what to do about grains. You could branch out. There's a whole other world of grains to explore. Some of these grains contain no gluten—brown rice, wild rice, quinoa, buckwheat, oats, millet, and amaranth—while others—barley, rye, spelt, and kamut—contain gluten but in much lower proportions than commercial wheat does.[28] Of course, if you have been diagnosed with celiac disease or have gluten sensitivity, you are limited to the no-gluten grains. Your local natural-foods stores usually offer breads made in small-scale and local bakeries using some of the above-listed grains. Pasta and breakfast cereals made from some of these grains are also becoming easier to find.

If you do choose wheat, try eating it less often and at least make it organic whole wheat, preferably made from sprouted grain, as found in a few brands of bread such as Manna Organics, Silver Hills Bakery, and Food for Life Baking Company's Ezekiel 4:9 bread. (These brands also offer breads made from a range of other sprouted whole grains.) Better yet, seek out ancient or heritage varieties of wheat. Spelt and kamut, a.k.a. khorasan, are ancient varieties belonging to the family of heritage wheat and are fortunately becoming increasingly available to the consumer. You can go more ancient still by searching for the earliest known wheat varieties—einkorn (never hybridized) or emmer, which date from as early as about ten thousand years ago. These "oldies" are very low-gluten grains and are sometimes well tolerated by those with a wheat allergy or sensitivity. Ancient wheat has had a much more straightforward history than that of conventional wheat, but it (particularly einkorn and emmer) is much less readily available. Some smaller farms across North America and around the globe continue to grow (or have started growing) these original "pre-Big Food" wheat varieties. Farmers' markets often supply consumers with bread or other products made from heritage wheat varieties (and other grain) grown in their region. I highly recommend these locally grown and produced heritage grain products. They're worth the search and the money! Producing these crops is good for Mother Nature, and consuming them is good for our health.

Note: All wheat contains gluten, although the amount differs depending on the variety.

Also note: While gluten sensitivity and celiac disease are certainly on the rise, and gluten is now increasingly avoided by those with whom it disagrees, bear in mind that gluten-free food does not necessarily equal healthy food. If gluten is a problem, always read your labels in order to avoid foods also high in sugar, hazardous fats, additives, preservatives, and food colorings.

As consumer demand has increased, you can now find more alternative grain products in mainstream stores as well as in the "old faithful" natural-food stores. Still, we can't always rely on the packaging claims to clearly reveal what's really inside. For example, "rye bread" or "ancient grains bread" may actually be found, upon a little closer inspection of the listed ingredients, to contain conventional wheat.

True Story

> Sarah, in her thirties, found that when she eliminated wheat from her diet, she very quickly knocked off those long-term saddle bags! Her other major symptoms—puffy, swollen fingers and ankles—also vanished. Fortunately, she was able to find other grains that agreed with her and that she also liked. Now, if Sarah occasionally eats a wheat product the puffiness will return and linger for a couple of days. At least she now knows why.

It's not uncommon to hear great health-improvement stories from people who have given up wheat altogether. They report relief from some of the following health problems and symptoms: migraines, depression, thyroid problems, chronic diarrhea, high blood pressure, acid reflux, insomnia, skin conditions, digestive pain, bloating, and obesity. Diabetics may also report improvement. Sometimes gluten is the problem and therefore the gluten-containing grains (mentioned above) must be avoided.

In my opinion, a lot of people would find it worthwhile to avoid conventional wheat for a six-week or longer trial. Then, perhaps at a different time, they could avoid all gluten-containing grains for a similar length of time. They would then be able to draw a personal conclusion about the difference that avoidance makes to their own health and general well-being.

Eating is an agricultural act.—Wendell Berry

Moving on to dairy: Some people find weight loss much easier if they cut out dairy. There are a number of different schools of thought among nutritional enthusiasts and experts today about the topic of dairy. One view (helpful in explaining the concerns around dairy consumption and the relation to weight gain and various health problems) is as follows: Your body may not have what it takes to adequately digest this product. Cow's milk, produced by herbivore female cows to nurse and nourish their own young, contains all the nutrients and naturally occurring hormones intended for calf growth and health. Given that human nutrient needs are much lower than those of a baby cow, cow's milk contains nutrients far in excess of the human body's processing ability.[29]

Another view says that people all over the world have been drinking milk from various animals, including cows, for thousands of years as an important source of nutrition. Surely these people knew what they were doing, so why would people today not do the same?

Whatever you decide on this issue is up to you, but for those who think drinking milk is the natural thing to do, here are a few points to consider.

Yes, people in cultures past usually knew intuitively what they were doing food-wise with what was available to them. However, they were until quite recently (if drinking cow's milk) consuming the real thing—real dairy—before industry got involved with it.

Today's dairy reality is a completely different story. By the time most dairy reaches your grocery store, it may contain antibiotics and chemical growth hormones*,[30] commonly used in the conventional dairy industry, and it has undergone artificial homogenization as well as pasteurization, a process that unfortunately destroys most if not all of the enzymes necessary for proper digestion.[31]

And my guess is that in preindustrial and pre–television-commercial times, people didn't think they needed to consume such massive amounts of dairy—regularly chugging down carton after carton of the stuff—in order to ensure that skeletal structures wouldn't crumble and that kids would grow. These fears have been implanted over several decades, thanks to the dairy industry's effective marketing campaigns and national food guides. It's obviously political.

It's quite likely that before pasteurization, in particular, but also before all the other chemical additions, and back when the standard dairy cow ate grass rather than a grain-based diet that includes corn, soy, and a range of mystery ingredients, and back when intuition and moderation dictated consumption, there wouldn't have been the health or weight problems that have now come to be associated with dairy.

Once again it comes down to quality and quantity. Can the body digest it, and if not, what then? Storage and other trouble! And on that note . . .

What about calcium, you ask? Isn't the reason we *need* to drink milk all about its calcium, which is commonly known to be so essential for bone health? Well, if so, then here's the deal. Milk does contain plenty of calcium, no doubt about it. That you already knew. What you may not know is that, despite the very high content of calcium in dairy, this calcium is not in a form that is readily absorbable by the human body.[32] Nutrients from food are only absorbed according

---

* Artificial Bovine Growth Hormone (rBGH, rBST) is legal for use in the US dairy cattle industry, but its use is prohibited in Canada (although Canada does allow imported BGH dairy milk and products from the United States). The entire European Union prohibits its use.

to how well your body can digest them. The fact of the matter is, once dairy is pasteurized, it can be very difficult to digest. If you're not digesting dairy well, then its calcium probably won't make it into your bones. When calcium is not deposited in its proper location, it can end up depositing itself throughout the body, in the arteries, joints, and kidneys, just to mention a few common places.[33] This is why today's high-dairy diets are associated with heart disease, arthritis, and kidney stones. If you eat a whole-foods diet with a good range of legumes, seeds and nuts, vegetables and fruit, you should be getting all the calcium and other nutrients your body requires. For extra calcium and other minerals (essential to calcium absorption) you can introduce soup-bone broths and seaweed into your diet.

In North America we tend to address deficiency with simple addition. If you are deficient in calcium, just consume more. That's pretty logical, but in calcium's case, we also need to hold on to it. Many foods and substances act to deplete calcium in the body, and therefore, even if you're consuming high amounts of this mineral, you may still be prone to deficiency and its associated conditions, such as osteoporosis. These depleting factors include caffeine, alcohol, high meat consumption, carbonated drinks, and junk food. Stress, tobacco, and prescription drugs can also interfere with mineral uptake and therefore interfere with keeping calcium in the bones.[34]

Fat-free dairy products are double trouble for calcium seekers because we all need the fat in dairy to help us absorb the calcium.[35]

True Story

Anne, a client I had several years ago, was crippled by intestinal and joint pain. She also experienced constant disappointment with her weight and had been constipated ever since she could remember. She agreed to try cutting out dairy. For her the difference was dramatic and seemed miraculous. She could not believe how much better her joints and bowels soon felt and functioned. She was also thrilled to gain control of her weight.

Also True

My mother was raised on a farm, drinking cow's milk provided by her family's own dairy cow. She went on to consume a moderate amount of dairy products throughout her life, but, by age sixty-five, she had developed osteoporosis. A childhood friend of hers has a worse story to tell. She grew up on a dairy farm, consuming plenty of dairy, but was diagnosed with advanced osteoporosis by the time she was fifty. Lifelong access to dairy is not always an osteoporosis preventive.

Something else to consider is that more and more studies are drawing a link between dairy consumption and hormone-related cancers, particularly breast[36] and prostate cancers.[37]

Still, I'm not suggesting that everyone cut out dairy, unless consuming it is causing some kind of physical trouble or discomfort. I'm simply offering some food for thought. Additionally, you might want to develop a backup plan aimed at osteoporosis prevention.

What I am suggesting, however, is that if you do decide that dairy is for you, try to make it the same wholesome dairy that people consumed back in the days of old. In other words, at least choose organic, free-range, drug-free, and preferably raw* milk (unpasteurized, with its full enzyme content). You may live in an area where raw dairy products can legally be sold in grocery stores, or else you may wish to find a good free-range dairy farm connection from which to buy your raw milk. Growing numbers of people today are searching for and choosing raw milk. They consider this milk to be an important part of their nourishment, bringing many health benefits (especially when fermented). They also find that bacteria risks associated with raw milk and other dairy products are not a problem when the milk is from a reputable organic, free-range, or grass-fed source. Some people are even members of dairy cow co-ops.

Note: Yogurt and other cultured/fermented dairy products, such as kefir and buttermilk, are easier to digest than regular milk because the culture and fermentation process has already helped to break them down.

Alternatives to cow's milk include goat's milk* almond milk, rice milk, hemp milk, coconut milk, and quinoa milk. These are found in most grocery stores. Be sure you purchase the unsweetened milk alternatives, because the "original" or vanilla or chocolate options usually contain a large amount of sugar.

Isn't it weird that we drink milk, stuff designed to nourish baby cows? How did that happen? Did some cattleman once say, "Oh, man, I can't wait till them calves are done so I can get me a hit of that stuff?"—Jerry Seinfeld

---

* Selling raw milk to the public is legal in just over half the United States and in most of Europe, although it is illegal in Canada.[38-40]

* Goat's milk possesses properties that more closely resemble those in human milk. It is also naturally homogenized and is often both better tolerated and easier to digest than cow's milk.[41]

True Story

Justin, now in his midtwenties, has had to avoid wheat and dairy since he was a child. Eczema, stomach aches, abnormal bowel movements, trouble focusing in class, and chubbiness were all common in his early years. When wheat and dairy were eliminated from his diet, his overall health improved dramatically. In no time, his grades went up, and his weight went down. Justin's mother found that he tolerated goat's milk and any of the alternate grains, making them fairly easy substitutes. He can now get away with the occasional consumption of wheat or diary without any symptoms recurring, but he most often chooses from the range of alternatives in order to remain trouble-free.

Note: Although wheat and dairy are two of the most common offenders because they have been overly tampered with and overeaten, almost any food is capable of causing a reaction or intolerance. Even some of the most nutritious foods may be bothersome if the digestive system can't manage to produce all that's necessary to break them down. For one person this food could be a certain grain and for another it could be a bean or a vegetable. For me, the only obvious offender is quinoa. How odd is that? I used to be able to eat it without incident, and I only ate it occasionally. But for the past few years, if I eat even a spoonful of quinoa, I quickly become sick with nausea, stomach ache, fatigue, weakness, and labored breathing. This is a blatant sensitivity, and because I know the offender I can most often easily avoid it. But for some, trying to find the actual culprit(s) responsible for the range of possible discomforts can be much more difficult. Each of us possesses a unique system that can change as we pass through different life stages. So seek to pinpoint the foods that bother you in any way and avoid them. A couple of months of strict avoidance of a bothersome food can sometimes result in a tolerance to it when you try it again. If this is the case, then reintroduced foods should be eaten only sparingly. Sometimes the intolerance is more lasting or even permanent.

Also note: Digestive differences between individuals may result from factors such as prescription drug use, lack of enzymes and/or healthful bacteria, poor diet/wrong foods, past or existing illness or disease, or malabsorption. Additionally, there may be genetically related biochemical differences that we were just born with. Several of these factors may be remedied or improved by following some of the tips in this book.

Tip #10

EAT ONLY WHEN HUNGRY AND ONLY ENOUGH TO FEEL SATISFIED

Waiting until you're actually hungry before you eat meals is a good policy for weight loss. When you wait, allowing for some hunger to grow, your body is given a window of time in which to convert back (to energy) and use up stored calories (fat) to supply its energy needs. Start thinking of a peckish episode as a good opportunity for a little weight loss as well as some much needed house-cleaning, the minicleanse, mentioned in Tip #5. Just add some water, and lemon if you wish, and let the internal clean-up begin.

Although it is important to eat only when hungry, try not to get to the point of being starving! Typically, the times we eat the foods we know we shouldn't eat occur when we've gone past the point of peckish and on to the "I could eat an entire pizza" type of hunger. It's a fine balance. Keep yourself satisfied and be aware of your hunger cues.

Note: When you do sometimes get too peckish or discover you can't last until lunch or dinner, you've found a perfect time to eat fruit because fruit is cleansing and can usually help tide you over.

Also note: If you are diabetic or experience low-blood-sugar challenges, be sure to consult your health-care provider to determine an appropriate eating schedule best suited to your individual blood-sugar needs.

Naturally, meal skipping can lead to all sorts of overeating and poor food choices—so don't skip meals. Eat only at mealtimes, whether you follow the standard three-meal (plus a snack or two, if necessary) approach to eating, or the five smaller meals preferred by some.

When mealtime finally does roll around, be sure to eat a sensible portion of food. If you eat until you're stuffed, you usually have more intake than your body can efficiently deal with. The digestive tract will be overworked and bogged down, and the unused calories will be stored as fat. Try to eat to the point where you feel 80 percent full. Wait about fifteen minutes, and if you're still hungry, eat a bit more. Usually by this time, though, your stomach will have sent a message to your brain that you are full enough.

Helpful hint: While your plate is still empty, try to determine with your head instead of your hunger how much food you will realistically need to put on that plate, just to be satisfied. Then stick to it. Exceptions are (a) you realize you've taken too much (then leave some) or (b) you feel you need more (then make it vegetables or a green salad).

> *When engaged in eating, the brain should be the servant of the stomach.*—Agatha Christie

True Story

Nicole, a high-school student, asked for my advice on healthy weight loss. She knew girls who already had eating disorders, and although she desired to lose weight, she wanted to learn how to achieve the loss in a healthy way. She admitted to skipping lunch and then eating a bag of chips or cookies after school. By this time she was so ravenous that she easily went overboard, inhaling one cookie after the next. I let her know that it is important to eat a healthy breakfast and then a nutritious lunch. This way she won't feel the strong desire to go hog wild on the junk food after school. She'll also be able to prevent the cycle of cravings and mood swings and the extra weight that the regular junk-food servings ensure. A nutritious breakfast and lunch will provide her with essential nutrients while giving her brain and body the fuel it needs to get her through the day well. I told her that the mass servings of junk food contain many more calories than her body can possibly use and that unless she was planning to run a marathon after consuming the junk food, the unused energy will both store as fat *and* leave her void of vital nutrients. I suggested that during those times when the temptation of cookies and chips was staring her in the face and she was watching her friends diving in, she could consider the novel idea of taking one cookie, eating it slowly, and enjoying it thoroughly. She could try limiting herself to one or two cookies or just a small handful of chips if total avoidance was impossibly difficult and unrealistic for her teenaged self to achieve. (This is a good exercise for almost anyone and need not be limited to teenagers.)

Her mother got on board with the revised menu and offered healthy snacks after school, including veggies with hummus, fruit, trail mix, or a light serving of tortilla chips with salsa and guacamole. She then followed with the same nourishing dinners that she had served previously. But the family now went without dessert, and they all tried not to eat past dinner. Nicole liked herbal tea with a little honey, and she enjoyed a cup of it in the evening as a comforting beverage or after school at the coffee shop, where she substituted it for the 350-calorie mochaccino. I encouraged her to walk home from school more often or do other physical activities that she enjoys a few times a week, thus speeding up her weight loss and doing wonders for her mind, mood, and health. During the weeks that followed she noticed that in addition to achieving some weight loss, she also had more energy, less extreme moods, and less acne (which was a big bonus).

Success is the sum of small efforts repeated day in and day out.—Robert J. Collier

Bonus Tip

HOW'S YOUR THYROID GLAND?

On a final note, if you have given your best effort, tried everything, and weight loss still comes slowly or not at all, you may want to consider a visit to your doctor's or naturopathic physician's office to have your thyroid gland function checked. Pronounced abdominal weight can be the result of an underactive thyroid. Remember that the thyroid is responsible for regulating your metabolic rate. And when the thyroid is imbalanced, the adrenals (the stress-fighting glands) also lack balance, so best get them checked too.[42] Symptoms of an underactive thyroid include distinct fatigue or lethargy, cold hands or feet, easy weight gain, inability to lose weight, unhealthy/dry/dull hair, flaky/dry/rough skin, mood swings, stiff feeling after sitting, high cholesterol, constipation, low pulse rate, low body temperature, and diminished sex drive.

Note: Any of the above symptoms can have different causes, not necessarily thyroid related, but if you are experiencing pronounced abdominal weight combined with several of the above-listed symptoms, it could be because of an underactive thyroid. A visit to your doctor is advisable.

Lastly, if you are one of those who struggle with weight gain caused by emotionally driven eating, you may benefit from the help of a qualified professional such as a counselor or psychologist. They can help detect and address the underlying reason(s) for overusing food for feel-good or coping purposes.

Checklist

23 DIFFERENT THINGS YOU CAN DO

Now that you've completed *Top Ten Best-Ever Healthy Weight-Loss Tips*, review the checklist below to set your goals. Check off any of the actions you've already begun to take and any of those you feel comfortable with and interested in committing to. For an effective weight-loss plan, you should check off a minimum of ten to twelve, and *exercise* should be one of them. Next, use the 21-Day Food/Weight/Fitness Journal to help you stay focused and motivated.

o Practice food combining (eat fruits alone and have proteins away from starches).

o Eliminate refined grains (replace with whole grains).

o Eliminate desserts and refined sugar (replace with natural sweeteners).

o Chew your food thoroughly.

o Increase enzymes (in your meals and/or by means of a supplement).

o Eliminate deep-fried foods and bad fats and oils (replace with healthy fats and oils in moderation).

o Drink warm lemon water in the morning.

o Increase fresh produce intake (going heavy on the leafy greens).

o Avoid alcohol.

o Reduce stress.

o Increase fiber.

o Take probiotics (via fermented foods or a supplement).

o Increase your water intake.

o Avoid empty calories.

o   Exercise (cardio and muscle building).
o   Reduce meat consumption (replace with plant-based protein sources).
o   Eat only grass-fed, organic, free-range meats.
o   Reduce or avoid dairy.
o   Reduce or avoid wheat.
o   Avoid foods that cause problems.
o   Eat only when hungry.
o   Stop eating when 80 percent full.
o   Get a sufficient amount of rest and sleep.

21-DAY FOOD/WEIGHT/FITNESS JOURNAL

Here are some suggestions for using this weight-loss, health, good habit, and change journal: The idea behind the 21-day aspect of this journal is to create a habit, whether it is to break old bad habits or begin new life-enhancing ones. In this journal you can keep track of all the food you eat or the food you plan to eat. Record how different foods make you feel when you eat them or when you avoid them. How do you feel after meals? Or at the end of a day? Or at the end of a week? Keep track of how everything you try makes you feel as you create new healthy habits like chewing, walking, or skipping dessert and get rid of old unhealthy habits like not chewing, being sedentary, or eating donuts. Also note any other improvements (e.g., to your skin, hair, mental condition, energy level, or quality of sleep) that result from making positive changes. Each page will offer you encouragement or reminders and other quotes or tips. As you transition to a new diet, old habits may rear their ugly heads, and you may have slip-ups. This is to be expected and, very importantly, should not result in self-judgment and a guilt spiral that first sends you into the "oh well, I'm off the wagon" mind-set, which in turn sends you to the bottom of an Oreo bag. Use these slip-up moments for information. Determine what led you here. Was it mood, energy, a missing dietary component, etc.? Record how you felt then.

I know the price of success: dedication, hard work,
and an unremitting devotion to the things you
want to see happen.—Frank Lloyd Wright

DAY 1

Helpful hint: To help remind yourself to chew more, create and post a "chew your food" card in the center of your table.

Thanksgiving dinners take eighteen hours to prepare. They are consumed in twelve minutes. Half-times take twelve minutes. This is not a coincidence.—Erma Bombeck

DAY 2

Try to eat your meals in a calm environment where there is minimal stress or distraction and without rushing. Then relax and breathe while you eat. All of these will help your meal to digest better, encouraging healthy weight.

_____

_____

_____

_____

_____

_____

_____

_____

_____

_____

The secret to staying young is to live honestly, eat slowly, and lie about your age.—Lucille Ball

DAY 3

If your job or your day is primarily a sedentary one, try to get out for a brisk fresh-air walk on one of your breaks. Walking will improve your digestion and burn off part of your lunch while enhancing your mental state and boosting your immune system, helping to ward off illness.

_____

_____

_____

_____

_____

_____

_____

_____

_____

_____

If it weren't for the fact that the TV set and the refrigerator are so far apart, some of us wouldn't get any exercise at all.—Joey Adams

DAY 4

Another good reason to drink the warm water with fresh-squeezed lemon juice is that it's an alkalizing beverage. Remember, a more alkaline diet is conducive to weight loss, whereas a more acidic diet is not. Vegetables are also very alkalizing (the greener, the better), and they are warriors in the fight for a healthy bacterial intestinal environment—a weight-loss and good-health wonderland.

_____

_____

_____

_____

_____

_____

_____

_____

_____

Insanity: Doing the same thing over and over again and expecting different results.—Albert Einstein

DAY 5

Want to lose weight sooner? Stay out of the fridge and cupboards between meals, especially if you've got high-calorie, poor-quality treats in there. Better yet, don't let those rascals in the house.

Cindy, a middle-aged mom, couldn't lose weight until her daughter started college and moved out of the house. With her went the cakes and ice cream that her mom found impossible to resist. Cindy lost eight pounds in one month by avoiding her daughter's desserts.

_____

_____

_____

_____

_____

_____

_____

_____

_____

A diet is the penalty we pay for exceeding the feed limit.—Unknown

DAY 6

Don't skip breakfast! Instead, why not switch over to cooked oats, spelt, or quinoa for breakfast? It will fill you up and boost energy, sustain blood-sugar levels, reduce midmorning cravings, and improve bowel function.

_____

_____

_____

_____

_____

_____

_____

_____

_____

_____

I used to skip breakfast, but eating gets my metabolism going, so I burn more calories all day.—Kate Walsh

DAY 7

Did you know that when we gobble down our food we often take in too much air, leading to belching, indigestion, and flatulence? Not cool! Slowing down and chewing food well actually helps prevent this sort of embarrassment and discomfort. Now that's cool! By now you've probably discovered it for yourself.

Don't delay, chew more today!

_____

_____

_____

_____

_____

_____

_____

_____

The past is a foreign country; they do things differently there.—Leslie Poles Hartley

DAY 8

Sinfully delicious desserts are little more than delayed disappointment. Does anyone really feel better after a piece of triple-layer chocolate cake? Sure, you feel incredible just up until the very last bite, then it's gone. Gone, gone, all gone, except for the guilt and the weight. Save yourself the disappointment and get into the habit of always saying no, until you reach your goal.

_____

_____

_____

_____

_____

_____

_____

_____

_____

_____

What you eat in private will show up in public.—Unknown

DAY 9

Are you getting enough sleep? Everything in your body functions better with sufficient sleep, including digestion, metabolism, appearance, bowels, and willpower. Being tired usually affects your mood and energy level, making it all the more tempting to consume a donut, chocolate bar, or ice cream in order to temporarily perk up your mind and put pep in your step. Say yes to sleep and you'll have the willpower to say no to the treat.

_____

_____

_____

_____

_____

_____

_____

_____

_____

_____

It's not that some people have willpower and some don't; it's that some people are ready to change and others are not.—James Gordon

DAY 10

Something else sleep-related—try not to eat dinner too late. Your body will still be in the process of digesting your meal well into the night when it really should be in a deep sleep. And you burn calories much faster when you're up and at it. Sleep time is for restoration and rejuvenation, not for working off a meal.

_____

_____

_____

_____

_____

_____

_____

_____

_____

_____

_____

*If I'm not good to myself, how can I expect
anyone else to be?—Maya Angelou*

DAY 11

Pile on the greens to reduce cravings. It turns out that when you increase your intake of veggies, particularly greens, you greatly boost your nutrients (e.g., vitamins, minerals, antioxidants, and EFAs). These keep your body not only healthier but also more satisfied, more energetic, less lacking, and less craving for something to help it feel better.

_____

_____

_____

_____

_____

_____

_____

_____

_____

_____

Life expectancy would grow by leaps and bounds if green vegetables smelled as good as bacon.—Doug Larson

DAY 12

Another reason to eat more greens, reds, oranges, and all the other colors of the rainbow, aside from how packed with vital nutrients they are, is that more energy/calories are required to digest them than are even contained in them. Celery is famous for this. You come out on the winning side when you load up on veggies.

_____

_____

_____

_____

_____

_____

_____

_____

_____

For all things produced in a garden, whether of salads or fruits, a poor man will eat better that has one of his own, than a rich man that has none.—J. C. Loudon

DAY 13

Portion Control—Part 1: Portion control is one of the keys for weight loss and also for longevity. When you eat too much (or too quickly) your body has to keep working harder and longer, and this overwork causes it to wear out sooner. You come factory-equipped with only one digestive system to last a lifetime, no spare parts. It's wise to show it a little respect and look after what you've been given by not overworking it.

_____

_____

_____

_____

_____

_____

_____

_____

_____

_____

My doctor told me to stop having intimate dinners for four,
unless there are three other people.—Orson Welles

DAY 14

Portion Control—Part 2: When deciding what to put in your body for each portion, think quality. Make your choices count! Your body parts will last even longer if they're well-maintained and fed the food that nature intended for human sustenance and vigor.

_____

_____

_____

_____

_____

_____

_____

_____

_____

_____

_____

*If I'd known I was going to live this long, I'd have
taken better care of myself.—Eubie Blake*

DAY 15

Portion Control—Part 3: Eat only when hungry. Eat only enough to feel satisfied—never stuffed. Eat real food. Follow these three rules and weight problems are unlikely.

_____

_____

_____

_____

_____

_____

_____

_____

_____

_____

_____

_____

I am a better person when I have less on my plate.—Elizabeth Gilbert, Eat Pray Love

DAY 16

We are what we eat, but we are also what we believe. Believe you're worth it—worth being healthy, feeling good, looking good, and achieving your ideal weight. Most of all, believe it's possible! You've only got this one life, for goodness' sake! Don't delay! Believe today!

_____

_____

_____

_____

_____

_____

_____

_____

_____

_____

First thing every morning before you arise, say out loud, "I believe," three times.—Norman Vincent Peale

DAY 17

Calorie counting is a relatively new concept. For most of history, no one knew what a calorie was; it hadn't been discovered yet. People didn't need to know because they just had real food, the real thing, homemade and hardly ever too much of it. Plus, they usually kept physically busy during the day, so they didn't need to know what exercise was, either. Calorie counting or burning off calories would have seemed absurd.

_____

_____

_____

_____

_____

_____

_____

_____

_____

_____

I never count calories, but I eat so well.—Alicia Silverstone

DAY 18

Get cooking! Spend more time preparing wholesome, homemade food in your kitchen where you're in control of ingredients. Eating out too often can mean too many hidden and mysterious ingredients, making for some unsolved weight-gain mysteries.

_____

_____

_____

_____

_____

_____

_____

_____

_____

_____

Eat to live, not live to eat.—Socrates

DAY 19

Don't skimp on quality, protein-rich foods. They keep us full (satisfied) longer and stabilize blood-sugar levels better. Too much protein, however (particularly animal protein), means a higher acidic environment (tough on kidneys), and loss of both calcium from bones and water from muscle. Too little protein prevents the good health of muscles, hair, nails, and almost everything else.

_____

_____

_____

_____

_____

_____

_____

_____

_____

To eat is a necessity, but to eat intelligently is an art.—François de La Rochefoucauld

DAY 20

Want to get high on life early in the day? Then work out early. It's a free, legal, natural, and good-for-you kind of high. Go ahead, make your day!

_____

_____

_____

_____

_____

_____

_____

_____

_____

_____

I have to exercise in the morning before my brain figures out what I'm doing.—Marsh Doble

DAY 21

Congratulations! For what? For whatever it was that you did to help reach your weight-loss goal and improve your health. Keep up the good work. And why not begin another 21-day habit now that you've come this far? You've already demonstrated to yourself what commitment can accomplish. Allow for flexibility as you continue to progress and learn, and refuse to be discouraged by any minor slip-ups that may happen along the way.

Be bold. Be confident. Be alive. A gallery of possibilities awaits you when you make change your friend.—Bob Bone

RECOMMENDED PACKAGED AND CANNED FOODS— NONPERISHABLE, REFRIGERATED, OR FROZEN

Amy's—soups, pizza, chili, frozen meals (enchiladas, lasagna, burgers, beans, Indian cuisine, Asian stir-fry)*, ** (some options are wheat-, gluten-, or dairy-free, and some are vegan)

Anita's Organic Mill—breakfast grain and seed mixtures*

Artesian Acres / Felicetti—kamut and spelt pasta

Artisana / Nuts To You / Once Again—nut and seed butters

Barbara's—fig, blueberry-fig, and raspberry-fig bars

Bubbies—lightly pasteurized sauerkraut, pickles

Ciao Bella / Sambazon—sorbet

Earth's Balance / Artisana—coconut oil/butter spread

Eden Foods—soups, rice and beans, beans, pasta sauce, tomatoes, kamut pasta, buckwheat soba noodles, whole-grain hot breakfast (rolled grains or flakes)

Emerald Valley Kitchen—salsa, humus, bean dip

Famous—falafel chips

Firefly Kitchens—unpasteurized kimchi, sauerkraut, and seasonal vegetables

Food for Life—Ezekiel 4:9 bread, Ezekiel 4:9 cereal, brown rice bread, brown rice tortillas*

Green & Black's / Camino / Endangered Species—organic/fair-trade dark chocolate

Imagine—soups

Karthein's Organic—unpasteurized sauerkraut

Late July—multigrain snack chips

Luna and Larry's Coconut Bliss / So Delicious—coconut ice cream

Lundberg—brown rice, brown basmati rice, brown jasmine rice, brown-rice chips
Manitoba Harvest—Hemp Bliss hemp milk, hemp seeds, hemp oil
Manna Bread—whole sprouted grain bread*
Mary's—crackers, pretzels, cookies
Natural Choice / Julie's Organic—frozen fruit bars
Nature's Path—breakfast cereal (hot and cold), granola, granola bars, waffles*
Pacific Foods—soups, hemp beverage
Prairie Market / Simply Natural—pasta sauce
Que Pasa—corn tortilla chips, corn tortillas, salsa
Rizopia / Tinkyada / Lundberg—brown-rice pasta
Ryvita / Wasa / Finn Crisp—rye crispbread
sardines/herring—canned (well drained)
Silver Hills—bread, bagels*
Silk Almondmilk
Simply Sprouted Way Better Snacks—black bean/multigrain/sweet potato chips
Stahlbush—frozen vegetables, beans, wild rice, rice and bean combo, fruit
Straus Family Creamery / Organic Meadows / Alden's—organic ice cream**
Suzie's Whole Grain Thin Cakes—brown rice, spelt and flaxseeds
Wholesome Sweeteners—molasses, coconut palm sugar, unrefined cane sugar, sucanat, date sugar, etc.
wild salmon—canned or frozen

Suggestions are based on considerations involving health-friendliness; weight-friendliness (exceptions—ice cream, chips); whole, unrefined ingredients; and sustainability concerns. Many of these products are vegan and, to the best of my knowledge, all products are without GMO ingredients. They are also wheat-free and dairy-free (with a few exceptions).*

---

*   Some products are wheat-free and gluten-free.

**   Contains dairy.

Many more healthy whole-food items (not mentioned here) are available in convenience packages at independent smaller or big natural-foods grocery stores or food co-ops in your area. Accessibility will vary depending on region, province, state, country, and store. Supporting local and smaller-scale producers is also a great idea—but wherever you go, read labels to ensure that quality/unrefined/natural ingredients are used.

Note: Some large natural-foods store chains carry their own labels (i.e., Whole Foods' 365 organic label and Trader Joe's own organic label). Items so labeled provide a good selection of products often produced with adherence to the above-listed concerns and considerations. They're also value priced. Just read the label.

When you go to the grocery store, you find that the cheapest calories are the ones that are going to make you the fattest—the added sugars and fats in processed foods.—Michael Pollan

A LIST OF RED-FLAG INGREDIENTS TO AVOID

Try to avoid ingestion of the artificial or chemically produced food additives that are potentially harmful to your health. Some additives can cause behavioral and neurological symptoms, while others are linked to cell mutation (tumor growth, cancer growth). These food additives can affect you in many adverse ways and produce such varied symptoms and reactions as migraine headaches, hyperactivity, anxiety, skin rashes, fatigue, mood changes, muscle cramping, visual disturbances, joint pain, sleep and breathing difficulties, etc. Listed below are some of the food additives to watch out for. For more information visit the sites that follow.

ammonium sulfate

Aspartame—also known as Nutra-Sweet and Equal

azodicarbonamide

brominated vegetable oil (BVO)

butylated hydroxyanisole (BHA) and butylated hydroxytoluene (BHT)

caramel coloring

carrageenan

food coloring—Blue #1 and #2, Red #3 and #40, FD&C Yellow #5 (a.k.a. tartrazine) and #6, Green #3

high-fructose corn syrup

monosodium glutamate/MSG (also called autolyzed vegetable protein, autolyzed plant protein, autolyzed yeast, yeast extract, natural flavoring, etc.)

nitrates and nitrites

olestra

partially hydrogenated vegetable oil

potassium bromate

saccharin

sodium benzoate

sulfites

List adapted from "Eat This, Not That," *15 Scariest Food Additives,* eatthis.menshealth.com/node/186430.

Also see these sites for more:

"Top 9 Scary Food Additives," ABC News, http://goo.gl /yQmKX.

"Top 10 Food Additives to Avoid," Mercola, http://goo.gl /WChAcH.

Visit the Environmental Working Group (EWG) at www.ewg .org for more information about choosing healthier consumer products. Also go to the Good Guide at www.goodguide.com for ratings of packaged food and other products, listed from healthiest to least healthy.

MORE ON ORGANIC, FAIR TRADE, LOCAL, AND GARDENING

Organic—In my opinion, the most important area in which to go organic is animal products, for the already-mentioned reasons—our health, animal health and welfare, and the planet. In addition to "organic," look for products labeled "local," "grass-fed," and "sustainable."

Otherwise, choose organic products where affordable, but remember that some foods are more contaminated by pesticides, herbicides, and other chemicals than others. You can access a list, updated each year by EWG (www.ewg.org), of the foods that are most and least heavily treated. With the "dirty dozen" (those most heavily treated), always buy organic. Don't worry about organic when it comes to the "clean fifteen" (those least heavily treated).

I find that a good organic sale can often be similar to or even lower in price than nonorganic. Look for third-party organic certification to ensure the item is truly organically grown. When it comes to organic produce, it is cheaper to buy when in season, which usually means local, too!

Other important and responsible agricultural methods used today are termed "biodynamic agriculture" and "sustainable agriculture."

Fair Trade—Fair trade items like chocolate (cocoa), bananas, and coffee are important to consider because not only are they sustainably grown but buying them also helps support and pay a fair price to small farms and their workers in the developing countries where these crops are grown.

Local—Buying locally grown products and shopping at local farmers' markets supports small farms and small-scale food manufacturers who use sustainable farming and manufacturing methods and minimal transportation for their products. Here you can also stock up and enjoy fresh and seasonal produce. Dining at local-food eateries is another great way to enjoy local goodness while showing your support.

Become a Gardener (if you haven't already done so)— Ever considered growing your own? Why not? Almost anyone can, and it's easy to learn how. There may even be a "vegetable gardening for beginners" workshop nearby or a community garden where you can join in with others. It will be the most organic, cheapest, freshest, most local food you can get. Fifty years ago, most households, whether in the city, suburbs, or country, relied on their own vegetable gardens to provide much of their produce. Fruit trees and berry bushes, even nut trees, were common in the yard. There is a growing trend to bring back the garden. Community gardens and patio or yard gardens are on the rise. To get your green thumb going, start with a few herbs, lettuce pots, or planter boxes and work your way up from there. Mother Nature and your own body will love you for it. Plus, you'll enjoy the other benefits: working with the earth to prepare the soil, planting the seeds, seeing them sprout and grow, and picking the harvest. All phases of gardening are good for the soul.

> *A garden was one of the few things in prison that one could control. To plant a seed, watch it grow, to tend it and then harvest it, offered a simple but enduring satisfaction. The sense of being the custodian of this small patch of earth offered a taste of freedom.*—Nelson Mandela

> *The first supermarket supposedly appeared on the American landscape in 1946. That is not very long ago. Until then, where was all the food? Dear folks, the food was in homes, gardens, local fields, and forests. It was near kitchens, near tables, near bedsides. It was in the pantry, the cellar, the backyard.*—Joel Salatin, *from* Folks, This Ain't Normal: A Farmer's Advice for Happier Hens, Healthier People, and a Better World

A FEW WORDS
CONCERNING GMOs

Something to think about in the midst of a big, controversial, politically charged debate: GMO stands for "Genetically Modified Organism." This refers to any organism (plant or animal) which has been altered at the gene level with the use of genetic engineering techniques. These include the transfer of genetic material from one species to another unrelated species. According to world-renowned geneticist and environmental activist David Suzuki, "GMO is bad science." He states that we are part of a massive scientific experiment and that it is too early to say that GMOs are safe because we don't yet know what the long-term consequences will be. The fact of the matter is that this industry is driven by money. GMO ingredients have been slipped into much of our food supply without any public discussion or awareness—they're ubiquitous —and our children are getting them in various products sold as children's foods. The consumer should be made aware of which foods are GMO and which products have GMO ingredients. To hear the full (brief) discussion, visit this link: http://goo.gl/puos4.

A recent Canadian study published in the scientific journal *Food and Chemical Toxicity*[43] shows that GM corn can cause severe negative health effects in laboratory rats fed GM corn compared to rats fed non-GM corn. These health effects included mammary tumors and kidney and liver damage, all leading to premature death.

An article appearing on the Healthy Home Economist blog* reveals a new study (2013) published in the scientific journal *Entropy* that connects GMOs and unexplained weight gain and other health problems. Find the article and a link to the study here: http://www.thehealthyhomeeconomist.com /roundup-quick-death-for-weeds-slow-and-painful-death-for-you/.

Perhaps the biggest problem associated with GMO foods is the lack of choice and awareness for the consumer. Despite multiple claims that GMO foods are safe to consume, corporate food companies and the US Food and Drug Administration have lobbied politically and financially to block laws that would require GMO foods to be labeled. Obviously, this makes it difficult to make informed decisions about the foods we buy and consume. A growing number of countries, including much of Europe, are choosing to label GMO foods. In 2013, the Connecticut legislature passed a law requiring GMO food labeling; the first such law to be passed in the United States. As of September 2013, legislation for GMO labeling was pending in at least 20 states in America.[44] No laws requiring GMO labeling have yet been passed in Canada. In some parts of the world there are outright bans on the sale and production of GMOs.

> *Biotechnology, variety patenting, and other agribusiness innovations are intended not to help farmers or consumers but to extend and prolong corporate control of the food economy; they will increase the cost of food, both economically and ecologically.*—Wendell Berry

Note: Your best assurance in purchasing non-GMO foods is to buy third-party certified organic or locally grown. Also look for "NON GMO Project" labeling. Cooking from scratch using whole foods—vegetables, grains, legumes, nuts and seeds,

---

* This blog is recommended for up-to-date information on many interesting and important topics including health and nutrition, our food supply, and sustainability concerns. You can follow it on Facebook.

organic/sustainable animal products—also greatly decreases exposure. This is because currently there are relatively few crops/ foods that are genetically modified; however, these GM crops are mass-grown and are estimated to have made their way into 80 percent of the food supply—processed, canned, packaged foods—and some are commonly used in livestock feed.

For a non-GMO shopping guide, go to www. nongmoshoppingguide.com. Here you will discover which foods are GMO, which ingredients are derived from GMO foods, and which products have GMO ingredients—including personal care products, supplements, and medicine.

To read more on GMO, see the following websites:

- www.foodandwaterwatch.org and

- www.organicconsumers.org.

Documentaries I recommend:

- *The Future of Food*

- *Genetic Roulette*

- *Food, Inc.*

> *Food, a Frenchman told me once, is the first wealth. Grow it right, and you feel insanely rich, no matter what you own.—Kristin Kimball*

CONCLUSION

By choosing to purchase good food and animal products and to live in a way that is weight-, health-, earth-, and animal-friendly, you can combat much of the harm created by modern agribusiness while preserving your own health. It's not too late to change the course of things for the future of our children and all generations to come.

The reality is that the consumer actually has the power to dictate what ends up on grocery store shelves. If it's not purchased, it will no longer be there. For example, if we decide we're not going to buy open-net farmed salmon or factory-farmed meat, those industries will shrivel or change their practices and methods of production. Power to change things is, as always, in the hands of the people.

Be the change you want to see in the world.—Gandhi

Thanks for taking the time to read these tips. I wish you great success with the weight loss and the improved health that will come as you explore the suggestions I have included here and apply the ones you personally find most relevant.

I invite you to contact me with your own true stories of weight loss and improved health resulting from following some of the tips provided in this book. With your permission, I may include some of them in my next book (in progress) on the topic of healthy whole-foods meal planning. This book will come complete with recipes, true stories, and more helpful weight-loss and digestive-health hints.

Please send your stories, if you wish, to tenbestever@gmail.com.

Visit my blog, *Elle's Top Health Tips* at http://ellestophealthtips. wordpress.com, for new and trending health topics and for updates on my ten tips. I'll be posting the latest discoveries and newest reports on the information I've shared with you here in this book, as well as more true stories.

May your good health increase and your weight loss endure!

NOTES

1. D. M. Sobieraj, S. M. Coleman, and C. I. Coleman, "U.S. Prevalence of Upper Gastrointestinal Symptoms: A Systemic Literature Review," *American Journal of Managed Care* 11 (2011): 449–58.
2. Patrick Holford, *Optimum Nutrition for the Mind* (California: Basic Health Publications, 2009), 17–25.
3. Miriam E. Bocarsly, Elyse S. Powell, Nicole M. Avena, and Bartley G. Hoebel, "High-Fructose Corn Syrup Causes Characteristic of Obesity in Rats: Increased Body Weight, Body Fat, and Triglyceride Levels," *Pharmacology Biochemistry and Behavior* (2010), doi: 10.1016/j.pbb.2010.02.012.
4. Joseph Mercola, "Artificial Sweeteners—More Dangerous than You Ever Imagined," *Mercola.com: Take Control of Your Health,* October 13, 2009, http://articles .mercola.com/sites/articles/archive/2009/10/13/artificial sweeteners-more-dangerous-than-you-ever-imagined .aspx.
5. David L. Katz, "Calories, Points, and Dots," *U.S. News and World Report,* July 8, 2013, http://health .usnews.com/health-news/blogs/eat-run/2013/07/08 /consider-the-quality-and-quantity-of-calories.
6. Udo Erasmus, *Choosing the Right Fats for Vibrant Health, Weight Loss, Energy, and Vitality* (Tennessee: Alive Books, 2001).
7. Cynthia Holzapfel and Laura Holzapfel, *Coconut Oil for Health and Beauty* (Tennessee: Healthy Living Publications, 2004).
8. Wolf Hamm and Richard J. Hamilton, *Edible Oil Processing* (England: Sheffield Academic Press, 2000).
9. Jane Higdon, "Chlorophyll and Chlorophyllin," Linus Pauling Institute—Micronutrient Center of Optimum

Health, 2005, http://lpi.oregonstate.edu/infocenter /phytochemicals/chlorophylls/#biological_activity.

10. Mark Hyman, *The Blood Sugar Solution* (New York: Little, Brown and Company, 2012).

11. Katy Cooper and Christine Hancock, "The Benefits of Regular Walking for Health, Wellbeing, and the Environment," *C3 Collaborating for Health,* 2009, http:// www.c3health.org/wp-content/uploads/2009/09/C3 -report-on-walking-v-1-20120911.pdf.

12. M. Irwin, A. Wilder, et al., "Influence of Pre- and Post-diagnosis Physical Activity on Mortality in Breast Cancer Survivors: The Health, Eating, Activity, and Lifestyle Study," *Journal of Clinical Oncology* 26, no. 24 (2008): 3,958–64.

13. J. N. Morris and A. E. Hardman, "Walking to Health," *Sports Medicine* 23, no. 5 (1997): 306–32.

14. Jeffery Alexander, "The Role of Resistance Exercise in Weight Loss," *Strength and Conditioning Journal* 24, no.1 (2002): 65–69.

15. Susan M. Kleiner and Maggie Greenwood-Robinson, *High Performance Nutrition: The Total Eating Plan to Maximize Your Workout* (New York: John Wiley & Sons, 1996).

16. N. D. Barnard, G. Turner-McGrievy, et al., "The Effects of Low-Fat, Plant-Based Dietary Intervention on Body Weight, Metabolism, and Insulin Sensitivity," *The American Journal of Medicine* 18, no. 9 (2005): 991–97.

17. Christopher Vasey, *The Acid-Alkaline Diet for Optimum Health* (Vermont: Healing Arts Press, 2006).

18. Y. Tantamango-Bartley, K. Jaceldo-Siegl, J. Fan, and G. Fraser, "Vegetarian Diets and the Incidence of Cancer in a Low-Risk Population," *Cancer Epidemiology Biomarkers and Prevention* 22, no. 2 (2013): 286–94.

19. P. Pitchford, *Healing with Whole Foods: Asian Traditions and Modern Nutrition* (California: North Atlantic Books, 2002), 507–8.

20. S. Barnes, "The Biochemistry, Chemistry, and Physiology of the Isoflavones in Soybeans and Their Food Products," *Lymphatic Research and Biology* 8, no. 1 (2010): 89–98.
21. S. Fallon and M. Enig, "Tragedy and Hype: The Third International Soy Symposium," *Nexus Magazine* 7, no. 3 (2000).
22. Jane Plant, *Your Life in Your Hands: Understand, Prevent, and Overcome Breast Cancer and Ovarian Cancer* (England: Virgin Publishing Ltd., 2001).
23. Daniel Doerge and Daniel Sheehan, "Goitrogenic and Estrogenic Activity of Soy Isoflavones," *Environmental Health Perspectives* 110, no. 3 (2002): 349–53.
24. Jen Gerson, "We're Farming in a Polluted World: Even Organic Foods Are Not GMO Free, Industry Leaders Say," *National Post,* February 13, 2013, http://news.nationalpost.com/2013/02/13/organic-foods-gm.
25. "Rearing Cattle Produces More Greenhouse Gas Gases Than Driving Cars, UN Report Warns," United Nations News Centre, November 29, 2006, www.un.org/apps/news/story.asp?newsID=20772#.UaaDipyrEhA.
26. Suzanne Goldenberg, "Eat Less Meat to Prevent Climate Disaster, Study Warns," *The Guardian,* April 13, 2012, http://www.guardian.co.uk/environment/2012/apr/13/less-meat-prevent-climate-change.
27. William Davis, *Wheat Belly* (New York: Rodale, 2011), 29.
28. Margaret M. Wittenberg, *The Essential Good Food Guide* (New York: Ten Speed Press, 2013).
29. Annemarie Colbin, *Food and Healing* (New York: Ballantine Books, 1986), 150.
30. "Bovine Somatotropin," *Wikipedia,* accessed May 29, 2013, http://en.wikipedia.org/wiki/Bovine_somatotropin.
31. Sally Fallon, *Nourishing Traditions* (Washington, DC: New Trends Publishing, 2001), 34–35.

32. Joel Fuhrman, *Eat to Live* (New York: Little, Brown and Company, 2011).
33. Annemarie Colbin, *Food and Healing*, 152.
34. Ibid., 160–62.
35. Annemarie Colbin, *The Whole Food Guide to Strong Bones: A Holistic Approach* (California: New Harbinger Publications, 2009), 89.
36. A. Hjartaker, P. Laake, and E. Lund, "Childhood and Adult Milk Consumption and Risk of Premenopausal Breast Cancer in a Cohort of 48,844 Women: The Norwegian Women and Cancer Study," *International Journal of Cancer* 93, no. 6 (2001): 888–93.
37. J. M. Chan, M. J. Stampfer, J. Ma, P. H. Gann, J. M. Gaziano, and E. Giovannucci, "Dairy Products, Calcium, and Prostate Cancer Risk in the Physicians' Health Study," *American Journal of Clinical Nutrition* 74, no. 4 (2001): 549–54.
38. "State-by-State Review of Raw Milk Laws," Farm to Consumer Legal Defense Fund, http://www.farmtoconsumer.org/raw_milk_map.htm.
39. "Raw Milk," *Wikipedia,* accessed May 12, 2013, http://en.wikipedia.org/wiki/Raw_milk.
40. "Statement from Health Canada About Drinking Raw Milk," Health Canada, http://www.hc-sc.gc.ca/fn-an/security/facts-faits/rawmilk-laitcru-eng.php.
41. "Goat Milk," The World's Healthiest Foods, accessed May 30, 2013, http://www.whfoods.com/genpage.php?tname=foodspice&dbid=131.
42. James M. Lowrance, *The Everything Adrenal Fatigue Book* (CreateSpace Independent Publishing Platform, 2010).
43. Gilles-Eric Séralini, Emilie Clair, Robin Mesnage, et al., "Long-term Toxicity of a Roundup Herbicide and a Roundup-tolerant Genetically Modified Maize," *Food and Chemical Toxicity* 50, no. 11 (2012): 4,221–31.

44. Stephanie Strom, "Connecticut Approves Labeling Genetically Modified Foods," The New York Times, June 3, 2013, http://www.nytimes.com/2013/06/04/business/connecticut-approves-qualified-genetic-labeling.html?_r=1&.